Chemistry and Applications of Green Tea

edited by

Takehiko Yamamoto, Ph.D.
Professor Emeritus
Osaka City University
Osaka, Japan

Lekh Raj Juneja, Ph.D.
Director (R&D)
Central Research Laboratories
Taiyo Kagaku Co., Ltd.
Yokkaichi, Mie, Japan

Djoing-Chi Chu, Ph.D.
Assistant General Manager
International Department
Taiyo Kagaku Co., Ltd.
Yokkaichi, Mie, Japan

Mujo Kim, Ph.D.
Managing Director (R&D)
Central Research Laboratories
Taiyo Kagaku Co., Ltd.
Yokkaichi, Mie, Japan

CRC Press
Boca Raton   New York

Acquiring Editor: Marsha Baker
Project Editor: Debbie Didier
Cover design: Dawn Boyd

Library of Congress Cataloging-in-Publication Data

Chemistry and applications of green tea / edited by Takehiko Yamamoto
    . . . [et al.].
        p. cm.
    Includes bibliographical references and index.
    ISBN 0-8493-4006-3
        1. Tea--Therapeutic use--Testing.   2. Plant polyphenols--
    Therapeutic use--Testing.   3. Tea--Composition.   I. Yamamoto,
    Takehiko.
        [DNLM: 1. Tea--chemistry.   2. Tea--metabolism.   3. Catechin--
    analogs & derivatives.   4. Catechin--pharmacology.   5. Catechin--
    therapeutic use.   WB 438 C517 1997]
    RM251.C355   1997
    615'.323624--dc21
    DNLM/DLC
    for Library of Congress   97-11614
                                                                    CIP

This book contains information obtained from authentic and highly regarded sources. Reprinted material is quoted with permission, and sources are indicated. A wide variety of references are listed. Reasonable efforts have been made to publish reliable data and information, but the author and the publisher cannot assume responsibility for the validity of all materials or for the consequences of their use.

Neither this book nor any part may be reproduced or transmitted in any form or by any means, electronic or mechanical, including photocopying, microfilming, and recording, or by any information storage or retrieval system, without prior permission in writing from the publisher.

All rights reserved. Authorization to photocopy items for internal or personal use, or the personal or internal use of specific clients, may be granted by CRC Press LLC, provided that $.50 per page photocopied is paid directly to Copyright Clearance Center, 27 Congress Street, Salem, MA 01970 USA. The fee code for users of the Transactional Reporting Service is ISBN 0-8493-4006-3/97/$0.00+$.50. The fee is subject to change without notice. For organizations that have been granted a photocopy license by the CCC, a separate system of payment has been arranged.

The consent of CRC Press LLC does not extend to copying for general distribution, for promotion, for creating new works, or for resale. Specific permission must be obtained in writing from CRC Press LLC for such copying.

Direct all inquiries to CRC Press LLC, 2000 Corporate Blvd., N.W., Boca Raton, Florida 33431.

© 1997 by CRC Press LLC

No claim to original U.S. Government works
International Standard Book Number 0-8493-4006-3
Library of Congress Card Number 97-11614
Printed in the United States of America 1 2 3 4 5 6 7 8 9 0
Printed on acid-free paper

EDITORIAL BOARD

Chairman	Takehiko Yamamoto	Osaka City University
Editors	Lekh Raj Juneja	Central Research Laboratories Taiyo Kagaku Co., Ltd.
	Djoing-Chi Chu	Central Research Laboratories Taiyo Kagaku Co., Ltd.
	Mujo Kim	Central Research Laboratories Taiyo Kagaku Co., Ltd.

Board Office Central Research Laboratories
Taiyo Kagaku Co., Ltd.
1-3 Takaramachi, Yokkaichi
510 Japan
Tel: +81-593-47-5400
Fax: +81-593-47-5417

CONTRIBUTORS

Djoing-Chi Chu, Ph.D.
Assistant General Manager
International Division
Taiyo Kagaku Co., Ltd., Japan

Hidehisa Takahashi, Ph.D. [a]
Manager
Central Research Laboratories
Taiyo Kagaku Co., Ltd., Japan

Kanari Kobayashi
Researcher
Central Research Laboratories
Taiyo Kagaku Co., Ltd., Japan

Laura Unten
Researcher
Central Research Laboratories
Taiyo Kagaku Co., Ltd., Japan

Lekh R. Juneja, Ph.D.
Director
Central Research Laboratories
Taiyo Kagaku Co., Ltd., Japan

Mamoru Koketsu, Ph.D. [b]
Group Leader
Central Research Laboratories
Taiyo Kagaku Co., Ltd., Japan

Manabu Ninomiya, Ph.D.
Group Leader
Central Research Laboratories
Taiyo Kagaku Co., Ltd., Japan

Masaaki Hibino
Group Leader
Central Research Laboratories
Taiyo Kagaku Co., Ltd., Japan

Masaki Matsumoto
Group Leader
Central Research Laboratories
Taiyo Kagaku Co., Ltd., Japan

Mitsuharu Masuda
Group Leader
Central Research Laboratories
Taiyo Kagaku Co., Ltd., Japan

Mujo Kim, Ph.D.
Managing Director
Central Research Laboratories
Taiyo Kagaku Co., Ltd., Japan

Noriyuki Ishihara
Group Leader
Central Research Laboratories
Taiyo Kagaku Co., Ltd., Japan

Senji Sakanaka, Ph.D.
Manager
Central Research Laboratories
Taiyo Kagaku Co., Ltd., Japan

Shigemitsu Akachi, Ph.D.
Assistant Manager
Central Research Laboratories
Taiyo Kagaku Co., Ltd., Japan

Takehiko Yamamoto, Ph.D.
Professor Emeritus
Osaka City University, Japan

Tsutomu Okubo
Assistant Manager
Central Research Laboratories
Taiyo Kagaku Co., Ltd., Japan

Present Address
[a] Coki Co., Ltd.
[b] Gifu University

PREFACE

Tea (tea infusion) is now one of the most popular drinks in the world, and its consumption nearly ranks with that of coffee. There are three kinds of tea: black tea, oo-long tea, and green tea. Their consumption as well as their manufacture, however, have been developed rather diverting into several regions of the world, respectively, though the tea trees for tea manufacturing belong to the same species taxonomically classified as *Camellia sinensis*, only that this species is further divided into two varieties of *assamica* (black tea) and *sinensis* (oo-long and green tea).

Tea was transferred from China to Japan in the early 8th century and used as a medicine. In the 15th century, green tea was used as a drink among the people of certain social strata and the manner of drinking tea was formulated in a special way which had to be mastered by so-called cultured men. Since the late 16th century, the custom of drinking tea infusion has been extended widely in civil society. This custom of drinking tea infusion became a daily necessity, and a word, "Nichijo sa han ji," was originated, which means that making cooked rice and green tea infusion are a routine work in our daily life (Nichijo, daily; sa, tea; han, cooked rice; and ji, to prepare and take).

Tea leaf is characterized as containing theanine (γ-aminoethylglutamic acid) as well as caffeine. Theanine is distributed only in tea trees and in buds of certain other *Camellia* sp. among various plants. Theanine is known to act as an antagonist of caffeine. On the other hand, a substantially different chemical composition is observed among the three teas because of the difference in their manufacturing processes. Green tea has the largest quantity of polyphenols of low molecular weights, especially of epigallocatechingallate ((-)-EGCg), epigallocatechin ((-)EGC), and epicatechingallate ((-)ECG) in decreasing order. This is because, unlike black tea and oo-long tea, green tea leaves used for manufacturing tea, are steamed immediately after harvesting to inactivate the enzymes which degrade above polyphenols in the leaf tissue.

The catechin derivatives described above are generally oxidizable on exposure to atmospheric oxygen, especially at alkaline sides. Also, they react with amino or thiol groups in the presence of dissolved oxygen. Recently, the polyphenols have been reported to act as a radical scavenger. The fact that green tea polyphenols are used as antioxidative material to protect from decolorization of carotene or from formation of rancidity in fat and oil is due to the chemical properties of tea polyphenols.

A great number of papers have been published on chemical components and the chemical properties of black tea, oo-long tea, and green tea. Also, there have been many papers published on the pharmaceutical effects or biochemical activities of those teas or their chemical components using various microorganisms or experimental animals. Recently, an arranged book titled *Chemistry and Function of Green Tea, Black Tea and Oo-long Tea* (in Japanese) was published by Nakabayashi, T., Ito, K., and Sakata, K. (1991) from Kagaku

Press Co., Ltd., Kawasaki, Japan.

Our research groups, together with several universities or institutes, have made efforts for the past 10 years in the developmental studies of several green tea components and discovered many interesting physiological, biochemical, and chemical activities or properties of those green tea components. Some of the results have been applied practically. Fortunately, this year is the 50 th anniversary of the Foundation of Taiyo Kagaku Co. Ltd., to which our Central Research Laboratories belong. To dedicate this anniversary, our research results published in various academic journals or authorized as patents are compiled by several editors and published as *Chemistry and Application of Green Tea* by the courtesy of CRC Press. We hope this book will be useful as a reference not only for researchers and engineers working in this field of tea science and manufacturing, but also for those in pharmaceutical science and chemistry of natural-occurring compounds. On this occasion, I would like to express my sincere thanks to Mr. Nagataka Yamazaki, President, and Mr. Yoshifumi Yamazaki, Vice president, of Taiyo Kagaku Co., Ltd. for their very positive support for publishing this book.

Takehiko Yamamoto, Ph. D.
Chairman of the Editorial Board

TABLE OF CONTENTS

CHAPTER 1
GREEN TEA - ITS CULTIVATION, PROCESSING OF THE LEAVES FOR
DRINKING MATERIALS, AND KINDS OF GREEN TEA
D.-C. CHU   1

CHAPTER 2
GENEREAL CHEMICAL COMPOSITION OF GREEN TEA AND ITS
INFUSION
D.-C. CHU AND L. R. JUNEJA   13

CHAPTER 3
CHEMICAL AND PHYSICOCHEMICAL PROPERTIES OF GREEN TEA
POLYPHENOLS
M. NINOMIYA, L. UNTEN, AND M. KIM   23

CHAPTER 4
ANTIOXIDATIVE ACTIVITY OF TEA POLYPHENOLS
M. KOKETSU   37

CHAPTER 5
METABOLISM OF TEA POLYPHENOLS
H. TAKAHASHI AND M. NINOMIYA   51

CHAPTER 6
CANCER CHEMOPREVENTION BY GREEN TEA POLYPHENOLS
M. KIM AND M. MASUDA   61

CHAPTER 7
SUPPRESSIVE EFFECT OF UREMIC TOXIN FORMATION BY TEA
POLYPHENOLS
S. SAKANAKA AND M. KIM   75

CHAPTER 8
GREEN TEA POLYPHENOLS FOR PREVENTION OF DENTAL CARIES
S. SAKANAKA   87

CHAPTER 9
INHIBITORY EFFECTS OF GREEN TEA POLYPHENOLS ON GROWTH AND CELLULAR ADHERENCE OF A PERIODONTAL DISEASE BACTERIUM, *PORPHYROMONAS GINGIVALIS*
S. SAKANAKA AND T. YAMAMOTO 103

CHAPTER 10
EFFECTS OF GREEN TEA POLYPHENOLS ON HUMAN INTESTINAL MICROFLORA
T. OKUBO AND L. R. JUNEJA 109

CHAPTER 11
DEODORIZING EFFECT OF GREEN TEA EXTRACTS
M. HIBINO AND S. SAKANAKA 123

CHAPTER 12
THEANINE - ITS SYNTHESIS, ISOLATION, AND PHYSIOLOGICAL ACTIVITY
D.-C. CHU, K. KOBAYASHI, L. R. JUNEJA, AND T. YAMAMOTO 129

CHAPTER 13
GREEN TEA EXTRACT AS A REMEDY FOR DIARRHEA IN FARM-RAISED CALVES
N. ISHIHARA AND S. AKACHI 137

TABLES OF DATA ON THE ANTIMICROBIAL ACTIVITIES OF GREEN TEA EXTRACTS
S. AKACHI, T. OKUBO, AND M. MATSUMOTO 145

INDEX 151

Chemistry and Applications of
of
Green Tea

Chapter 1

GREEN TEA - ITS CULTIVATION, PROCESSING OF THE LEAVES FOR DRINKING MATERIALS, AND KINDS OF GREEN TEA

D.-C. Chu

TABLE OF CONTENTS

I. Introduction
II. Origin and Cultivation of Tea Plants
   A. The Place of Origin and Characteristics of the Tea Plants
   B. Cultivation of Tea Plants and Utilization of Leaves
III. Processing of Green Tea Leaves
IV. Kinds of Green Tea
References

I. INTRODUCTION

The tea plant is a kind of evergreen laurel tree and is taxonomically classified as *Camellia sinensis* (L.) O. Kuntze of the family of *Theaceae*. The tea plant spontaneously grows widely from tropical to temperate regions in Asia and has been closely associated with people's life since the dawn of history. The content of caffeine, polyphenols, and theanine in the leaves of *C. sinensis* characterizes the taste of the tea infusion, and this species is distinguished from other related wild species (Table 1) [1, 2]. These characteristic chemical components in tea leaf must be the reason why tea has long been utilized and loved as one of the best beverages in the world up to now. People utilized the leaves or its infusion as a medicine at first and then, to make a luxury drink. At present the tea plant is cultivated in more than 20 countries of Asia, Africa, and South America as one of the most favorite horticultural plants just like coffee and cacao.

One of the most important processes in tea manufacturing for drink is fermentation. It is known that the conversion of tannin in tea leaves is not achieved by microorganisms but by enzymes present in the leaves, and so, this phenomenon should be called "enzymation," exactly. The degree of fermentation greatly affects the quality and type of tea. According to the degree of fermentation, tea is classified into green tea (unfermented), oo-long tea (semi-fermented), and black tea (fullyfermented).

In this chapter the place of origin of the tea plant, processing of tea leaves to obtain a material for drink, and general chemical composition of green tea leaves and its infusion are briefly described.

II. ORIGIN AND CULTIVATION OF TEA PLANTS

A. THE PLACE OF ORIGIN AND CHARACTERISTICS OF TEA PLANTS

Sealy elaborated a comprehensive research on the genus of *Camellia* dealing

Table 1
Contents of Several Characteristic Chemical Components in Leaves of Genus *Camellia* and Interspecific Hybrids
(g per 100 g dried leaves) [1, 2]

Species	Polyphenols*					Theanine	Caffeine
	(+)-C	EC	EGC	ECg	EGCg		
I. *Thea*							
C. sinensis							
var. *sinensis*	0.07	1.13	2.38	1.35	8.59	1.21	2.78
var. *assamica*	0.02	1.44	0.35	3.35	12.10	1.43	2.44
C. taliensis	tr.**	0.58	0.8	1.9	6.84	0.27	2.54
C. irrawadiensis	0.03	0.72	0.12	0.67	0.21	0.21	0
II. *Camellia*							
C. japonica							
var. *japonica*	0.25	4.81	0	0	0	0	0
var. *decumbens*	2.04	3.57	0	0	0	0	0
C. reticulata	0.11	0.26	0	0	0	0	0
C. saluenensis	0.07	0.35	0	0	0	0	0
C. pitardii	0.25	6.64	0.46	0	0	0	0
III. *Paracamellia*							
C. sasanqua	0	0.02	0	0	0	0	0
C. oleifera	0.19	0	0	0	0	0	0
C. kissi (seedling)	tr.**	tr.**	0	0	0	0	0.02
IV. Hybrids							
C. sasanqua × *C. sinensis*	0.22	0.23	0.07	0.29	0.56	0.05	2.48
C. sinensis × *C. japonica*	0.03	0.49	0.81	0.34	1.14	0.15	0.25
C. japonica × *C. kissi*	0	tr.	0	0	0	0	0

*(+)-C, catechin; EC, epicatechin; EGC, epigallocatechin; ECg, epicatechin gallate; EGCg, epigallocatechin gallate.
**tr.: trace

with more than 80 species for taxonomy in addition to the score previously reported [3]. He classified the genus *Camellia* into eight separate sections, of which *Thea* comprises five species: *C. sinensis, C. irrawadiensis, C. taliensis, C. grocilipes*, and *C. pubicosta*. The tea plants, being cultivated at present and economically evaluated, belong to the species of *Camellia sinensis* and are roughly classified into two varieties, *assamica and sinensis* (Table 2 and Plates 1 and 2 following page 36) [3-6]. Spontaneous growth of *C. sinensis* var. *assamica*, whose leaf is large (leaf length and width, 16 - 19 × 7 - 9 cm) and trunk is tall, are in the area ranging from Yun-nan province of China to the northern region of Myanmer and Assam region of India. On the other hand, that of var. *sinensis*, whose leaf is small (leaf length and width, 5.5 - 6.1 × 2.2 - 2.4 cm) and the trunk is bush type, are observed in the eastern and southeastern districts of China (Figure 1).

Table 2
Taxonomical Classification of Tea and Related Plants [3-6]

Watt (1907)	Cohen-Stuart (1919)	Kitamura (1950)	Sealy (1958)
Section *Thea*			
Camellia thea Link.	*C. theifera* (Griff.) Dyer	*C. sinensis* (L.) O. Kuntze	*C. sinensis* (L.) O. Kuntze
var. *bohea*	var. *bohea*	var. *sinensis*	var. *sinensis*
var. *stricta*			
var. *lasiocalyx*			form *parvifalia* (Mig.) Sealy
var. *viridis*			
Race			
1. Yunnan & China	var. *macrophylla*	form *macrophylla*	form *macrophylla* (Sieb.) Kitamura
2. Burma & Sham	var. *burmaensis*		
3. Assam Indigenus			
4. Lushai	var. *assamica*	var. *assamica*	var. *assamica* (Mast.) Kitamura
5. Nage Hills			
6. Manipur			

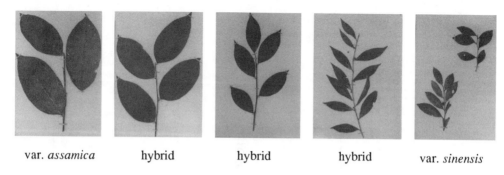

| var. *assamica* | hybrid | hybrid | hybrid | var. *sinensis* |

Figure 1. Leaf shapes of *Camellia sinensis*, var. *assamica*, var. *sinensis,* and the intraspecific hybrids. Various sizes and shapes of leaves are seen among the hybrids [5, 8, 9].

For a long time, botanists have asserted the dualism of tea origin from their observations that there exists distinct differences in the morphological characteristics between Assamese varieties and Chinese varieties [6, 7].

Hashimoto and Shimura reported that the differences in the morphological characteristics in tea plants are not necessarily the evidence of the dualism hypothesis from the researches using the statistical cluster analysis method [5, 8]. In recent investigations, it has also been made clear that both varieties have the same chromosome number (2n=30) and can be easily hybridized with each other. In addition, various types of intermediate hybrids or spontaneous polyploids of tea plants have been found in a wide area extending over the regions mentioned above. These facts may prove that the place of origin of *Camellia sinensis* is in the area including the northern part of the Myanmer, Yun-nan, and Si-chuan districts of China (Figure 2) [5, 9, 10-14]. This area is the cradle place of a characteristic agriculture which is named as the Culture of Lucidophyllus Forest [11,12]. Also this area is overlapped with a region which is presumed to be the original place of several cultivating crops [7, 13,14].

The fermentability (activity of polyphenol oxidase) and content of polyphenols in young tea leaves greatly differ depending on the kind of cultivars (cultivated varieties). Those cultivars which show better fermentability and higher content of polyphenols are evaluated to be a good quality for black tea manufacture. Almost all of the cultivars belonging to the var. *sinensis* group have relatively low fermentability and less content of polyphenols. The fermentability of tea leaves is genetically regulated as shown by the activity of polyphenol oxidase which is controlled by a polygene system, and its heritability shows a high value (0.6-0.9) [15]. Therefore, this genetic trait has been taken as one of the main marks in the breeding program of tea, especially of black tea.

Tea plants have been cultivated in a wide range from the Republic of Georgia in the north to New Zealand in the south. The area of cultivation of tea and the yield of tea leaves in Asia are far greater than other regions, amounting to about 82 (1993) and 87% (1994) of the world, respectively (Table 3) [16-18].

One of the most important factors for tea plant cultivation is tolerance to the cold. This genetic trait is controlled by a polygene system, and its heritability is nearly 0.9. This high value affords a wide adaptability of tea plants growing in a broad area from temperate to tropical regions. The cultivars of var. *sinensis* can survive in winter as cold as -12°C, whereas those of var. *assamica* perish at -4°C in a few weeks. Therefore, the former cultivars have been cultivated in the temperate regions and the latter in the tropical and subtropical regions. Almost all of the tea plants grown in Japan are of var. *sinensis* and are utilized for green tea preparation.

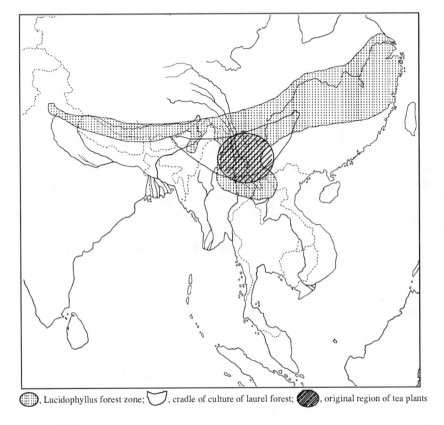

, Lucidophyllus forest zone; , cradle of culture of laurel forest; , original region of tea plants

Figure 2. The inferential region of the origin of tea plants [5, 9, 10-14].

Table 3

Production and Cultivation Area of Tea in the World [16-18]

Year Region	Production (×1,000 kg)				Cultivation Area (×1,000 ha)			
	1979-81	1991	1992	1993	1979-81	1991	1992	1993
Asia	1,476	2,074	2,010	2,152	2,021	2,114	2,138	2,269
Africa	202	339	298	341	169	206	205	211
South America	44	62	59	60	47	49	47	47
Oceanea	8	9	9	9	3	4	4	5
Others	129	120	59	83	80	77	74	73
World	1,859	2,604	2,435	2,645	2,320	2,450	2,468	2,605

B. CULTIVATION OF TEA PLANTS AND UTILIZATION OF LEAVES

The tea plant is a vegetatively propagated plant, and the propagation of tea plants is usually done by the cloning method. Although the seedling propagation method is rarely applied, the uniformity in the growth and characteristics of generated seedlings are scarcely seen because of their genetic heterogeneity. In three to four years after tea tree cuttings which were rooted on the nursery field and later transplanted to the farm, the young plants are pruned and arranged into a semicylindrical shape to be convenient for field work. Young buds and leaves of five-to-six year old trees are nipped three to four times a year. The yield of the first harvest (Ichiban cha) reaches 6,000 kg/ha, which is harvested in early summer and deals with the highest quality, the second (Niban cha), 5,000 kg/ha and the third (Sanban cha), 4,000 kg/ha in average. Thus, the total annual yield of tea leaves in Japan is about 15,000 kg/ha based on the fresh weight.

The tea plant contains various useful chemical compounds. People might have begun to eat it or drink its water extract as a medicine in ancient time. Even now, for example, Shan tribes in the Shan state of Myanmer utilize the tea leaves for making tea pickles known as Leppet tea, which is a fermentation product by microorganisms and eaten as a vegetable [9, 19]. The utilization of Leppet-type tea leaves is also observed in Miang in the northern part of Thailand and Nie-en in the Xishuang-banna region in the southern part of the Yun-nan district of China.

During a long historical time, the merit of tea as a physiologically functional agent or the habit of eating tea leaves has gone out gradually, and a preferential use of tea leaves as a drink has prevailed. Thus, skillful processing methods of the tea leaves suitable for each type of tea drinks have been established. Now, a great number of people enjoy drinking tea at their leisure time.

III. PROCESSING OF GREEN TEA LEAVES

The processed tea leaves are classified into three types according to the degree of fermentation-unfermented, semi-fermented, and fullyfermented tea leaves, and they are called green tea, oo-long tea, and black tea, respectively.

A distinctive feature of green tea processing is that the leaves are never subjected to the condition for causing fermentation. In the case of manufacture of green teas, the harvested fresh leaves are immediately steamed at 95-100°C for 30-45 sec. to inactivate the enzymes contained, especially polyphenol oxidase (Figure 3). The steaming treatment protects degradation of vitamins and thus, the content of vitamins in green tea is much higher than fermented teas (Table 4) [20, 21].

The steamed leaves are then rolled to make a slender pickle form followed by drying in current air of moderate temperature. The moisture content of fresh leaves that is usually 78-80%, decreases to about 10% during the rolling process. The rolling process disrupts the leaf tissue and mixes them uniformly in the shape as far as possible. The drying subsequently applied increases aroma and preservability of the products. The rolled and dried leaves called Aracha are finally fired (roasted) and cut to prepare the final products by tea dealers. The firing treatment is also important to remove the original coarse aroma and add a fired tea flavor [22].

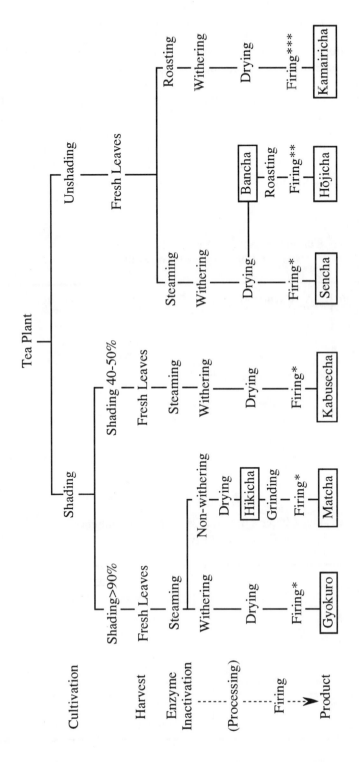

Figure 3. Processing of tea leaves and kinds of green tea products [20-22, 24]. Degree of firing to produce flavor: *, mild; **, considerably strong; ***, strong.

The decision of the suitable time for leaf harvesting and the growing techniques of tea plants seriously affect the quality of green tea, as well as the cultural and environmental conditions. The tea leaves harvested in the season of early summer are usually superior in quality to those harvested in later seasons (Table 5) [21, 24]. Shading of the tea plant increases the amount of amino acids, especially of theanine in young shoots, and decreases the polyphenol content. The price of green tea largely depends on the quality. There is a high correlation between the price of tea and content of amino acids, especially of theanine or arginine [23]. Correlation coefficients between the total score of sensory test and content of total nitrogen, theanine, and total free amino acids were estimated to be 0.91, 0.87, and 0.86, respectively [24]. The tea of highest quality, Gyokuro, for example, costs almost 10 times as much as the lower quality one, Ban-cha. For this reason, farmers of tea plantations in Japan make their efforts to produce the tea leaves of quality as high as possible (See Plate 3 following page 36).

Table 4

Contents of Several Vitamins in Tea Leaves
(mg per 100 g dry tea leaves) [20, 21]

Kinds of Tea \ Vitamin	A (Carotene)	B_1	B_2	Niacin	C
Matcha	28.9	0.6	1.35	4	60
Sencha	13	0.35	1.4	4	250
Bancha	14	0.25	1.4	5.4	150
Kamairicha	5.8	0.35	1.8	7	200
Oo-long Tea	28.3	0.13	0.86	5.7	43
Black Tea	17.4	0.1	0.8	10	32

Table 5

Seasonal Changes in Some Chemical Components of
Green Tea Leaves [21, 24]

Components	Harvested in	
	Early Summer	Late Summer
Soluble Fraction (%)	46.99	49.95
Polyphenols (%)	10.89	14.85
Total nitrogen (%)	5.31	4.52
Theanine (mg per 100 g leaves)	1,613	404
Caffeine (%)	3.07	3.48
Free amino acid (%)	1.9-3.2	0.5-1.0

IV. KINDS OF GREEN TEA

Most green tea leaves are utilized for making green tea infusion. The main components of green tea leaves and its infusion are shown in Table 6 [20, 21, 25, 26].

Among 100,000 tons of annual consumption of green tea in Japan, 78.6% of them are processed to produce Sencha, 12% Bancha, and 0.4% Gyokuro [24].

The production of Matcha, a specially ground Hikicha, is only 0.6% of total tea consumption. Despite its small consumption, Matcha keeps a very important situation historically and in Japanese culture. A man called "Sen no Rikyu" established a special manner of drinking tea for mental training in the era of Azuchi Momoyama (A.D.1573-1600). This manner of drinking tea, called as Cha-no-yu, has been succeeded up to date. Matcha is suspended into hot water, agitated well with a brush made of bamboo named Chasen, and served in the traditional way (See Plates 4 and 5 following page 36).

Tea leaf is rich in polyphenols and the amount is more than 10% on a dry basis. It is also rich in caffeine amounting to about 1 to 4% of the dried leaf. The content of amino acids, especially those of theanine and glutamic acid, are relatively high [26, 27]. These chemical components have various physiological functions which will be described in other chapters of this book.

Table 6

Some Chemical Components in Dried Tea Leaves
Depending on Their Quality [20, 21, 25, 26]

Kinds of Tea	Grade	Polyphenols (%)	Caffeine (%)	Theanine (mg/100g)	Free amino acids (mg/100g)	Total N (%)
Gyokuro	Medium	13.4	3.1	1,480	2,730	5.48
Matcha	High	6.5	3.85	2,260	5,800	6.36
	Medium	6.2	3.51	1,790	4,610	5.85
	Low	6.5	3.23	1,170	3,400	5.38
Sencha	High	14.7	2.87	1,280	2,700	5.48
	Medium	13.3	2.8	1,210	2,180	5.35
	Low	14.5	2.77	612	1,460	4.45
Bancha	Medium	12.45	2.02	N.A.	770	3.83
Hojicha	Medium	10.37	1.93	N.A.	200	3.46
Oolong	Medium	16.03	2.34	588	993	3.43

N.A., not analyzed

REFERENCES

1. **Nagata, T. and Sakai, S.,** Differences in caffeine, flavonols and amino acid contents in leaves of cultivated species of *Camellia, Jpn. J. Breed.,* **34**, 459, 1984.
2. **Nagata, T. and Sakai, S.,** Caffeine, flavonol and amino acid contents in leaves of hybrids and species of section *Dubial* in the genus *Camellia, Jpn. J. Breed.,* **35**, 1, 1985.
3. **Sealy, J. R.,** *A Revision of the Genus Camellia,* The Royal Horticultural Society, London, 1958.
4. **Kitamura, S.,** Tea and *Camellia (in Japanese), Shokubutsu-bunrui-chiri,* **14**, 297, 1950.
5. **Hashimoto, M. and Shimura, T.,** Morphological studies on the origin of the tea plant (V), *Jpn. J. Trop. Agr.,* **21**, 93, 1978.
6. **Cohen-Stuart, C. P.,** A basis for tea selection, *Bulletin du Jordin Botanique de Buitenzorg,* **1**, 193, 1919.
7. **Harler, C. R.,** *The Culture and Marketing of Tea,* Oxford University Press, London, 1964.
8. **Hashimoto, M. and Shimura, T.,** Morphological studies on the origin of the tea plant (IV), *Jpn. J. Trop. Agr.,* **20**, 1, 1976.
9. **Hashimoto, M.,** Searching origin of tea, in *A searching the Origin of Tea,* Tanko-sha, Kyoto, 1988, p 222.
10. **Chen, C. and Chen, Z. G.,** Yun-nan is the original place of tea plant, *Bull. An hui Province Agriculture College,* **26**, 1, 1978.
11. **Nakao, S.,** *Nature-It's Morphological Studies (in Japanese),* Morishita, M. and Kira, T., Eds., Chuo Koronsha, Tokyo, 1967.
12. **Sakai, K.,** *Before Rice Cultivation (in Japanese),* Nihon Hoso Shuppan Kyokai, Tokyo, 1971.
13. **De Candlle, L.,** *The Origin of Cultivated Plants (in Japanese),* Kamo, G., Trans., Iwanami-Shoten, Tokyo, 1953.
14. **Toyao, T.,** *Collection of gene resource of plants in Japan (in Japanese),* Matsuo, T., Ed., Kodan-sha, Tokyo, 1989.
15. **Toyao, T.,** Varietal difference and breeding behavior of fermentation ability (polyphenol oxidase activity) in tea plants, *Jpn. Agr. Res. Quart.,* **18**, 37, 1984.
16. **FAO,** *Production Year Book,* **47**, 174, 1993.
17. **FAO,** *Quart. Bull. Stat.,* **7**, 29, 1994.
18. **FAO,** *Quart. Bull. Stat.,* **8**, 18, 1995.
19. **Eden, T.,** *Tea,* Longmans, London, 1958.
20. **Standard Tables of Food Composition in Japan** (in Japanese), Resources council, Science and Technology Agency, Tokyo, 1991.
21. **Yamanishi, T.,** *Encyclopedia of Food, Agriculture and Nutrition (in Japanese),* Kodan-sha, Tokyo, 1981.
22. **Hara, T.,** Studies on the firing aroma and off-flavor components of green tea, *Bull. Nat. Inst. Veg. Ornam. Tea,* **3**, 9, 1989.
23. **Mukai, T., Horie, H., and Goto, T.,** Differences in free amino acids and total nitrogen contents among various prices of green tea, *Tea Res. J.,* **76**, 45, 1992.
24. **Ohishi, S.,** *Development of Tea Manufacture in Japan (in Japanese),*

Nousangyoson Bunka Kyokai, Tokyo, 1983.
25. **Ikegaya, K.**, Determination of the content of total nitrogen, caffeine, total free amino acid, theanine and tannin of Sencha and Maccha by near infrared reflectance spectroscopy, *Bull. Nat. Res. Inst. Veg. Ornam. Tea*, **2**, 47, 1988.
26. **Shojaku, S., Takayanagi, H., Anan, T., and Ikegaya, K.**, Chemical composition of Chinese bai-cha, huang-cha, ging-cha and hei-cha and the preference test for the these teas, *Tea Res. J. (in Japanese)*, **60**, 59, 1984.
27. **Muramatsu, K.**, *Chemistry of Tea (in Japanese)*, Asakura Shoten, Tokyo, 1991.

Chapter 2

GENERAL CHEMICAL COMPOSITION OF GREEN TEA AND ITS INFUSION

D.-C. Chu and L. R. Juneja

TABLE OF CONTENTS

I. Introduction
II. Chemical Components of Green Tea
    A. Tea Polyphenols
    B. Caffeine
    C. Amino Acids and Other Nitrogenous Compounds
    D. Vitamins
    E. Inorganic Elements
    F. Others
        1. Carbohydrates
        2. Lipids
References

I. INTRODUCTION

An old Chinese book on pharmaceutical plants written in about 200 B.C. referred to the detoxification effect of the tea leaf. In the early 8th century, green tea was transferred to Japan from China for medicinal use. Green tea infusion gives specific taste and flavor, and it is now one of the most popular drinks in the world. The infusion is characterized as containing such compounds as tea polyphenols, caffeine, theanine, vitamins, etc. [1, 2].

The general chemical composition of the green tea leaf and its infusion are briefly described in this chapter.

II. CHEMICAL COMPONENTS OF GREEN TEA

As shown in Table 1, the largest component of green tea leaves is carbohydrates including cellulosic fiber and the next is protein, but these components are almost insoluble. Only the components of relatively small molecular weights which are infused with hot water give a specific accent to the tea infusion [3].

A. TEA POLYPHENOLS

One of the noticeable components of green tea leaves is so-called tea polyphenols which are almost infused with hot water or extracted with ethyl acetate from the aqueous solution. The slight astringent and bitter taste of green tea infusion is attributed to the polyphenols. The contents of green tea polyphenols which are composed of six kinds of catechin and its derivatives slightly deviate depending on the species of tea plant and the season for harvesting, as shown in Table 2 [4-7, 28]. (-)-EGCg is the largest and next to this are (-)-EGC, (-)-ECg, (-)-EC in the decreasing order in amount.

Table 1
General Chemical Components of Tea Leaves and its Infusion (per 100 g) [1-3]

Kinds of Tea		Moisture (g)	Protein (g)	Lipid (g)	Carbohydrates		Ash (g)	Minerals (mg)					Vitamins						Caffeine (%)	Tannin (%)
					Sugar (g)	Fiber (g)		Ca	P	Fe	Na	K	A (U)	A (IU)	B1 (mg)	B2 (mg)	Niacin (mg)	C (mg)		
Gyokuro	leaf	3.1	29.1	4.1	32.7	11.1	6.4	390	410	10.4	11	2,800	21,000	12,000	0.30	1.16	6.0	110	3.5	10.0
	infusion*	98.6	0.7	0	tr.**	0	0.3	2	12	0.1	1	180	0	0	0.01	0.06	0.3	10	0.16	0.23
Matcha		4.8	30.7	5.3	28.6	10.0	7.4	420	350	17.0	6	2,700	29,000	16,000	0.60	1.35	4.0	60	3.2	10.0
Sencha	leaf	4.9	24.0	4.6	35.2	10.6	5.4	440	280	20.0	3	2,200	13,000	7,200	0.35	1.40	4.0	250	2.3	13.0
	infusion*	99.6	0.1	0	0.1	0	0.1	2	1	0.1	2	18	0	0	0	0.03	0.1	4	0.02	0.07
Kamairicha	leaf	5.0	24.2	3.5	35.6	10.7	5.5	490	250	24.0	4	2,200	13,000	7,200	0.35	1.80	7.0	200	2.5	13.0
	infusion*	99.7	0.1	0	0	0	0.1	3	1	tr.**	1	22	0	0	0	0.03	0.1	3	0.01	0.05
Bancha	leaf	4.4	19.7	4.4	33.5	19.5	5.5	740	210	38.0	4	1,900	14,000	7,800	0.25	1.40	5.4	150	2.0	11.0
	infusion*	99.8	tr.**	0	tr.**	0	0.1	3	1	0.1	1	21	0	0	0	0.02	0.1	2	0.01	0.03
Hojicha	leaf	2.2	18.2	4.8	39.2	18.7	5.5	490	280	12.9	6	1,900	12,000	6,700	0.10	0.82	5.6	44	1.9	9.5
	infusion*	99.8	tr.**	0	tr.**	0	0.1	2	2	tr.**	1	24	0	0	0	0.02	0.1	tr.**	0.02	0.04
Oo-long Tea	leaf	5.4	19.4	2.8	39.8	12.4	5.3	310	230	32.4	7	1,800	15,000	8,300	0.13	0.86	5.7	8	2.4	12.5
	infusion*	99.8	tr.**	0	tr.**	0	0.1	2	1	tr.**	1	13	0	0	0	0.03	0.1	0	0.02	0.03
Black Tea	leaf	6.0	20.6	2.5	32.1	10.9	5.2	470	320	17.4	3	2,000	900	500	0.10	0.80	10.0	0	2.7	20.0
	infusion*	99.4	0.2	0	0.1	0	0.1	2	3	0	2	16	0	0	0	0.01	0.2	0	0.05	0.10

* Infusion preparation: 3 g of ground leaves were soaked in 100 ml of boiling water for 2 min., and the extract was analyzed.
**tr.: trace

(+)-GC and (+)-C are usually trace or a minor component. The ester type catechins, (-)-ECg and (-)-EGCg are stronger in bitterness and more astringent than (-)-EC and (-)-EGC.

Catechin is synthesized in tea leaves through malonic acid- and shikimic acid-metabolic pathways. Gallic acid is derived from an intermediary product produced in the shikimic acid-metabolic pathway (Figure 1).

A number of papers have been published on the antimutagenic activity [8-11], suppressive effect of chromosome aberration [12], antioxidant activity [13], depressor effect on renal hypertension [14], inhibitory effect on lipid peroxidation [15], or inhibitory effects on arteriosclerosis [16, 17] of green tea polyphenols [18].

Physiological and functional activities of tea polyphenols will be mentioned in detail in several chapters of this book. Also, the structures and chemical and physicochemical properties of green tea polyphenols will be described in the following chapter.

Table 2

Seasonal Change and Differences in Contents of Polyphenols Depending on Tea Species (g per 100 g dried leaves) [4-7, 28]

Polyphenols		var. *sinensis*		var. *assamica*	*C. tariensis*	*C. irrawadiensis*
		Spring	Summer			
(+)-Catechin	(C)	tr.*	0.07	0.02	—	—
(+)-Gallocatechin	(GC)	tr.*	tr.*	—	—	—
(-)-Epicatechin	(EC)	1.50	1.50	1.13	0.58	0.76
(-)-Epicatechin gallate	(ECg)	2.80	4.10	3.35	1.90	0.75
(-)-Epigallocatechin	(EGC)	4.00	3.70	0.35	0.80	0.12
(-)-Epigallocatechin gallate	(EGCg)	8.80	12.20	12.10	6.84	0.25

*tr.: trace

B. CAFFEINE

The plant species which contain caffeine are few, but most of the caffeine-containing plants have been utilized as favorite foods or beverages since ancient times.

Caffeine is a trimethyl derivative of purine 2, 6-diol (Figure 2) and is synthesized mainly in leaves of the tea plant. Occurrence of caffeine was first observed in coffee by Runge in 1820. Nakabayashi isolated a similar compound from tea and named it theine [4]. Later, caffeine and theine were identified to be the same compound. The caffeine content of coffee beans is usually 1.5%, while that of green tea leaves reaches 5% at the maximum. Caffeine is also found in maté leaves (*Ilex paraguariensis*, Paraguay tea, 0.2-2%), cacao paste (*Theobroma cacao* 0.3%) and cola nuts (*Cola nitida* 1-2%). The content of caffeine is generally high in the tea leaves evaluated as high quality by sensory test.

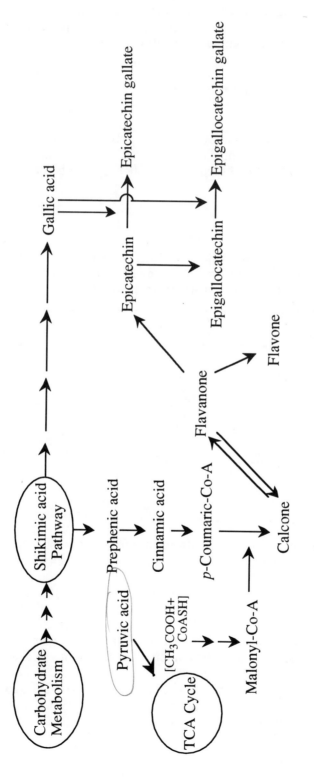

Figure 1. Biosynthetic pathway of catechins in tea plant [4].

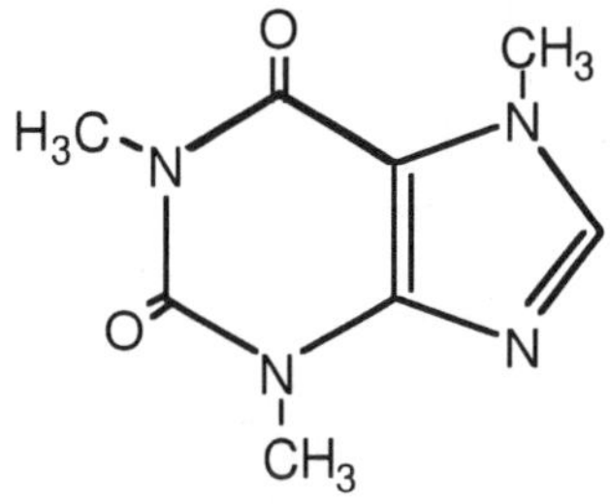

Figure 2. Chemical structure of caffeine.

Caffeine has been applied as a cardiac stimulant and a diuretic. It also stimulates the cerebral cortex to induce excitation in the central nervous system. On the other hand, it causes irritation of the gastrointestinal tract and sleepless for certain people. For these reasons, various methods have been suggested to remove caffeine. Almost all of these methods, however, were not practically effective because of unavoidable contamination of organic solvents [19-25].

We found that a cyclodextrin-polymer helps removing caffeine specifically filtrate among various components in green tea infusion (Figure 3). The β-cyclodextrin polymer was the most effective to separate caffeine among α-, β- and γ-cyclodextrins or their polymers. When an infusion of tea is applied on the column of the β-cyclodextrin polymer, only caffeine passes through the column while tea polyphenols are adsorbed on the column and eluted with 30-50% ethanol. A problem of this method is that at present no good method of preparing an effective β-cyclodextrin polymer have been known, except using epichlorohydrin for polymerization of the cyclodextrin.

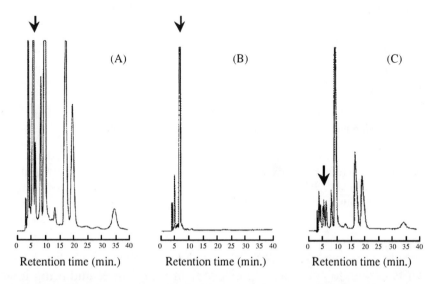

Figure 3. Liquid chromatograms of green tea infusion before and after filtration through a column of β-cyclodextrin-polymer. (A), Green tea infusion; (B), filtrate passed through a column of β-CD polymer; (C), eluates with 50% ethanol of the column used for filtration of green tea infusions. Arrow shows the peak of caffeine.

C. AMINO ACIDS AND OTHER NITROGENOUS COMPOUNDS

About one fifth of the total nitrogen found in green tea infusion originates from caffeine and related compounds. Other nitrogenous compounds in the tea infusion are amino acids, amides, certain proteins, and nucleic acids. Most of the proteins in tea leaves are insoluble because of binding with tannins that occurs during the process of green tea manufacturing.

The content of total nitrogen in green tea extract ranges from 4.5 to 6.0%, and about a half of it is of free amino acids. Theanine and glutamic acid are the major amino acids in the green tea infusion, and aspartic acid and arginine are the next (Table 3) [26, 27]. The contents of amino acids in tea leaves harvested in spring are larger than those harvested in later seasons [28, 29].

Theanine is a very unique amino acid and is known to be produced by the tea plant and certain species of genus *Camellia*. The rate of metabolism of theanine in tea leaves is slow, but its transport from root to leaf is so rapid that this amino acid is accumulated in tea leaves [30]. Chemical and biochemical characteristics of theanine are described in Chapter 12.

Table 3

Main Free Amino Acids in Green Tea Infusion [26, 27]

Amino acid	Range of Content	Average	Relative %
Theanine	194.0 - 2,771.5	1,201.9	45.9
Glutanic acid	154.5 - 441.1	277.2	12.7
Arginine	16.3 - 909.0	265.0	9.2
Aspartic acid	131.0 - 352.0	226.6	10.8
Glutamine	24.2 - 599.7	206.1	7.5
Serine	43.1 - 282.2	83.9	3.8
Threonine	16.5 - 80.9	30.4	1.4
Alanine	20.8 - 85.6	29.9	1.4
Asparagine	3.1 - 45.0	23.1	1.2
Lysin	5.4 - 42.2	21.2	1.0
Phenylalanine	7.4 - 38.6	20.8	1.1
Valine	4.6 - 137.2	19.8	1.0

60 samples were used for examination. Preparation of tea infusion: 100 g of hot water was added to 100 mg of ground dry tea leaves, and the mixture was kept at 80°C for 30 min.

γ-aminobutyric acid (GABA) is found widely in animal and plant kingdoms. GABA is known to act as a suppressive neurotransmitter and bring lowering effect of blood pressure [31, 32]. Streeter and Thompson reported that GABA and alanine were accumulated in radish leaves under anaerobic conditions [33]. Tsushida and Murai also revealed that glutamic acid acts as a source of nitrogen for increasing the contents of GABA and alanine in tea leaves. They succeeded in obtaining a new type of green tea which contains GABA in high concentrations by treatment of tea trees with nitrogen gas and carbon dioxide gas. The infusion of the new green tea named as Gabaron tea was reported to show the preventive effect on increase of blood pressure [34].

D. VITAMINS

Commercial green tea leaves contain vitamin C (VC, ascorbic acid) of about 280 mg per 100 g dried leaves. But, the vitamin C content of oo-long tea or black tea is less than green tea, because it is decomposed during their fermentation process (Table 1).

A story tells us that green tea and semi-fermented tea were very effective for protecting crews from scurvy during their long cruise in the age of the Great Voyage in the 16-17th century. Thus, green tea became one of the most useful materials for sailors at that time.

E. INORGANIC ELEMENTS

Some specific inorganic compounds in the tea plant are aluminum, fluorine, and manganese (Table 4).

Table 4
Inorganic Elements and Their Contents in Green Tea Leaves
(per 100 g dried leaves) [3, 4]

Element	Content		Element	Content	
N	3.5-7.1	(g)	Al	420-3,500	(ppm)
P	0.2-0.7	"	As	0.20-0.42	"
K	1.6-2.5	"	Ba	1.3-5.1	"
Ca	0.12-0.57	"	Br	7.8-25.0	"
Mg	0.12-0.30	"	F	17-260	"
S	0.24-0.48	"	Na	20-33	"
Fe	100-200	(ppm)	Ni	1.3-5.9	"
Mn	500-3,000	"	Pb	2.2-6.3	"
Cu	15-20	"	Rb	8-44	"
Mo	0.4-0.7	"	Sc	0.2	"
B	20-30	"	Se	1.0-1.8	"

The levels of aluminum and fluorine in tea leaves are relatively higher than other plants. Tea plant is scarcely affected even in the field containing large amounts of aluminum sulfate which is a main causal factor of acidic soil. It has been presumed that the tea plant has a biochemical mechanism to neutralize the toxicity of aluminum. In the study by analysis with NMR, Nagata observed that in tea leaf aluminum exists mainly in a chelate form, indicating that catechins prevent the expression of damage by accumulation of aluminum. This finding may be one of the important physiological significances of tea polyphenols [35].

Fluorine has been known to show a preventing effect against dental caries. This element exists in tea leaf as anion. Fluoride anion produces various fluor compounds and covers the surface of teeth to prevent bacterial attack. The tea roasted at high temperatures contains an aluminum fluoride complex, but it may be ineffective against dental caries because of its inactivity.

F. OTHERS
1. Carbohydrates

The total carbohydrate contained in green tea leaves is about 40% and one third of it is cellulosic fiber (Table 1). Starch is also contained and affects the quality of green tea. The synthesis of starch begins with dawn and ends at sunset. Therefore, the content of starch in tea leaves varies significantly in a day. Starch in tea leaves harvested in the morning is less than that in the afternoon, and tea leaves harvested in the morning are usually evaluated to be better in quality.

2. Lipids

Tea leaves contain oil in average of 4% by weight. Tea seeds also contain oil of 20-35, 30-35, and 43-45% by weight in Japanese, Chinese, and Assam cultivars, respectively. The oil is nondrying, and its solidifying temperature is -5 to +15°C. The ratio of liquid fatty acid to solid is about 6.14 (Table 5). Tea seed oil is seldom utilized nowadays.

Tea plant has been widely utilized from the ancient age for its specific aroma, taste, or excellent physiological function. Pharmaceutical functions of chemical compounds and detailed analysis of these components have not been carried out for a long time.

Recently, effectiveness of many kinds of functional fractions like polyphenols or theanine have been revealed, and some of their functions are described in this book.

Table 5

Composition of Fatty Acids of Tea Seed Oil [3, 4]

Fatty acid			
Saturated fatty acid	14.0 (%)	Unsaturated fatty acid	86.0 (%)
Palmitic acid	75.1	Oleic acid	89.4
Stearic acid	8.5	Linoleic acid	10.6
Myristic acid	7.4		
Others	9.0		

REFERENCES

1. **Nagata, T. and Sakai, S.**, Caffeine, flavonol and amino acid contents in leaves of hybrids and species of section *Dubial* in the genus *Camellia*, *Jpn. J. Breed.*, **35**, 1, 1985.
2. **Nagata, T.**, Studies on useful components of tea in leaves of the genus *Camellia*, *Bull. Nat. Res. Inst. Tea 44 (in Japanese)*, **21**, 253, 1986.
3. **Standard Tables of Food Composition in Japan,** Resources Council, Science and Technology Agency, Tokyo, 1991.
4. **Nakabayashi, T.**, Chemical components in tea leaves, in *Chemistry and Function of Green Tea, Black Tea, and Oolong tea (in Japanese)*, Nakabayashi, T., Ina, K., and Sakata, K., Eds., Kogaku Shuppan, Kawasaki, Japan, 1991, p 20.
5. **Oshima, Y.**, Chemical studies on the tannin substance of formosan tea-leaves, *Bull. Agr. Chem. Soc. Japan*, **12**, 103, 1936.
6. **Bradfield, A. E., Penney, M., and Wright, W. B.**, The catechins of green tea. Part I, *J. Chem. Soc.*, 32, 1947.
7. **Bradfield, A. E. and Penney, M.**, The catechins of green tea. Part II, *J. Chem. Soc.*, 2249, 1948.
8. **Ruan, C., Liang, Y., Liu, J., Tu, W., and Liu, Z.**, Antimutagenic effect of eight natural foods on molsy foods in a high liver cancer incidence area, *Mutat. Res.*, **279**, 35, 1992.
9. **Wang, Z.-Y., Cheng, S. J., Zhou, Z. C., Athar, M., Khan, W. A., Bickers, K. R., and Mukhtar, H.**, Antimutagenic activity of green tea polyphenols, *Mutat. Res.*, **223**, 273, 1989.
10. **Kada, T., Kaneko, K., Matsuzaki, S., Matsuzaki, T., and Hara, Y.**, Detection and chemical identification of natural bio-antimutagens: a case of the green tea factor, *Mutat. Res.*, **150**, 127, 1985.
11. **Stich, H. F., Chan, P. K. L., and Rosin, M. P.**, Inhibitory effects on phenolics, teas, and saliva on the formation of mutagenic nitrosation products of salted fish, *Int. J. Cancer*, **30**, 719, 1982.
12. **Ito, Y., Ohnishi, S., and Fujie, K.**, Chromosome aberrations induced by aflatoxin B1 in rat bone marrow cells *in vivo* and their suppression by green tea, *Mutat. Res.*, **222**, 253, 1989.
13. **Yen, G. and Chen, H.**, Antioxidant activity of various tea extracts in relation to their antimutagenicity, *J. Agric. Food Chem.*, **43**, 27, 1995.
14. **Yokozawa, T., Oura, H., Sakanaka, S., Ishigaki, S., and Kim, M.**, Depressor effect of tannin in green tea on rats with renal hypertension, *Biosci. Biotech. Biochem.*, **58**, 855, 1994.
15. **Okuda, T., Kimura, Y., Yoshida, Y., Hatano, Y., Okuda, H., and Arichi, S.**, Studies on the activities of tannins and related compounds from medicinal plants and drugs. I. Inhibitory effects on lipid peroxidation in mitochondria and microsomes of liver, *Chem. Pharm. Bull.*, **31**, 1625, 1983.
16. **Kimura, Y., Okuda, H., Okuda, T., Yoshida, T., Hatano, T., and Arichi, S.**, Studies on the activities of tannins and related compounds from medicinal plants and drugs. II. Effects of various tannins and related compounds on adrenaline-induced lipolysis in fat cells (1), *Chem. Pharm. Bull*, **31**, 2497, 1983.

17. **Kimura, Y., Okuda, H., Okuda, T., Yoshida, Y., Hatano, T., and Arichi, S.**, Studies on the activities of tannins and related compounds from medicinal plants and drugs. III. Effects of various tannins and related compounds on adrenocorticotropic hormone-induced lipolysis and insulin-induced lipogenesis from glucose in fat cells (2), *Chem. Pharm. Bull*, **31**, 2501, 1983.
18. **Hara, Y., Matsuzaki, T., and Suzuki, T.,** Angiotensin I converting enzyme inhibiting activity of tea components, *Nippon Nogeikagaku Kaishi (in Japanese)*, **61**, 803, 1987.
19. **Barch, W. E.**, Decaffeination of coffee, *US patent* 2817588, 1957.
20. **Adler, I. L. and Earle, E. L., Jr.**, Process for preparing a decaffeinated soluble coffee extract, *US patent* 2933395, 1960.
21. **Van der Stegen, G. A.**, A process for removing caffeine and substances that are potentially detrimental to health from coffee, *European Patent* 0158381, 1985.
22. **Zeller, B. L., Kaleda, W. W., and Saleeb, F. Z.**, Coffee extract decaffeination method, *US patent* 4521438, 1985.
23. **Saleeb, F. Z. and Zeller, B. L.**, Roasted coffee extract deca, *US patent* 4547378, 1985.
24. **Jones, G. V., Meinhold, J. F., and Musto, J. A.**, Non-caffeine solids recovery process, *US patent* 4505940, 1985.
25. **Katz, S. N.**, Decaffeination process, *US patent* 4472442, 1984.
26. **Mukai, T., Horie, H., and Goto, T.**, Differences in free amino acids and total nitrogen contents among various prices of green tea, *Tea Res. J.*, **76**, 45, 1992.
27. **Ikegaya, K., Takayanagi, H., Anan, T., Iwamoto, M., Uozumi, J., Niahinari, K., and Cho, R.**, Determination of the content of total nitrogen, caffeine, total free amino acids, theanine and tannin of Sencha and Matcha by near infrared reflectance spectroscopy. Bulletin of the National Research Institute of Vegetables, *Ornamental Plants and Tea*, 47, 1988.
28. **Takeo, T.**, Formation of amino acids induced by ammonia application and seasonal level fluctuation of amino acid contents in tea plant, *Chagyogijutsu Kenkyu (in Japanese)*, **56**, 70, 1979.
29. **Mizuno T., Katayama, Y., and Funaki, T.**, Studies on the carbohydrates of tea. Part XI. The contents of starch in green leaves of tea, *Nisshokukoshi (in Japanese)*, **12**, 373, 1965.
30. **Takeo, T.**, Ammonium-type nitrogen assimilation in tea plants, *Agric. Biol. Chem.*, **44**, 2007, 1980.
31. **Shibata, S., Itokawa, S., Mikawa, U., Shoji, J., and Takido, M.**, *Yakuyo Tennennbutsu Kagaku (in Japanese)*, Nannzanndo, Tokyo, 1982.
32. **Stanton, H. C.**, Mode of action of gamma amino butyric acid on the cardiovascular system, *Arch. Int. Pharmacodyn.*, **143**, 195, 1963.
33. **Streeter, J. G. and Thompson, J. F.**, Anaerobic accumulation of γ-aminobutyric acid and alanine in radish leaves (*Raphanus sativus*), *Plant Physiol.*, **49**, 572, 1972.
34. **Tsushida, T.**, Clarification of amino acids metabolism in tea leaves and development of new type tea-Gabaron tea, *Tea Res. J.*, **72**, 43, 1990.
35. **Nagata, T.**, New analytical methods for studying tea quality components, *Tea Res. J.*, **72**, 53, 1990.

Chapter 3

CHEMICAL AND PHYSICOCHEMICAL PROPERTIES OF GREEN TEA POLYPHENOLS

M. Ninomiya, L. Unten, and M. Kim

TABLE OF CONTENTS

I. Introduction
II. Separation and Purification of Green Tea Polyphenols
    A. Preparation of Green Tea Polyphenols
    B. Separation and Purification of Green Tea Polyphenol Components
III. Chemical and Physicochemical Properties of Green Tea Polyphenols
IV. Recent Developments on Chemical and Physicochemical Properties of Polyphenols
    A. New Polyphenols Isolated from Green Tea Leaves
    B. Reactivity of Polyphenols to Various Substances
References

I. INTRODUCTION

The major tasty components of green tea infusion are polyphenols, caffeine, and several amino acids including theanine. The content of these components differ considerably depending on the species of tea plant, the soil for tea cultivation, and the method of processing tea leaves for manufacturing tea material. The ratio of these components greatly affect the flavor and taste of green tea infusion.

Polyphenols are produced as a secondary metabolite of higher plants. Plant polyphenols may be divided into two major groups: proanthocyanidins and the polyesters based on gallic acid and/or hexahydroxydiphenic acid and their derivatives [1]. Green tea polyphenols are a class of flavanols which are C15 compounds, and their derivatives are composed of two phenolic nuclei (A ring and B ring) connected by three carbon units (C-2, C-3, and C-4). The flavanol structure of catechin (3,3',4',5,7-pentahydroxyflavan) contains two asymmetric carbon atoms at C-2 and C-3. Green tea polyphenols which are readily extracted with ethylacetate are mainly composed of (+)-catechin, ((+)-C); (-)-epicatechin, ((-)-EC); (+)-gallocatechin, ((+)-GC); (-)-epigallocatechin, ((-)-EGC); (-)-epicatechin gallate, ((-)-ECg); (-)-gallocatechin gallate, ((-)-GCg); and (-)-epigallocatechin gallate, ((-)-EGCg). Catechin and its derivatives also have nucleophilic centers at C-6 and C-8 which are reactive with electrophilic specimens. They are highly chemically reactive, showing the properties of metal chelator, oxidative radicals scavenger, nitrosation inhibitor, etc.

The chemical, physicochemical, and biochemical studies of the green tea polyphenols have been performed by many researchers for some decades.

Various reports about the chemical and physicochemical properties have been increased by the development of analytical techniques such as nuclear magnetic resonance (NMR), mass spectrometry (MS), and several other analytical methods including high performance liquid chromatography, recycling liquid chromatography, etc. Intensive investigations have been carried out especially on (-)-EGCg, and its physiological functions have been well documented [2-4].

It is known that polyphenols form several complexes in the reaction with caffeine [5, 6], proteins and peptides [7], metal ions [8], or cyclodextrins [5]. In the presence of dissolved oxygen, it is highly likely that the chemical properties of the forming complexes of green tea polyphenols with the substances mentioned above are closely related to the physiological functions of green tea polyphenols.

This chapter presents: 1) A method of purification, isolation, and identification of each component of ethylacetate soluble polyphenols of green tea leaves and 2) several data on chemical and physicochemical properties of each of the components reported so far by many researchers which will be necessary or useful for the scientists and engineers who are studying or working in the field of plant chemistry, or pharmaceutical and food science and in their applications.

II. SEPARATION AND PURIFICATION OF GREEN TEA POLYPHENOLS

A. PREPARATION OF GREEN TEA POLYPHENOLS

Green tea leaves were steeped into 10 weights of hot water at 95°C for 30 min with gentle stirring. The mixture was pressed, the juice was filtered, and the filtrate was concentrated to about a quarter by volume *in vacuo*. The water extract was partitioned with an equal volume of ethylacetate three times, and the ethylacetate layer was brought to dryness *in vacuo* and used as green tea polyphenols ("SUNPHENON^R," a commercial preparation, Taiyo Kagaku Co., Ltd.).

B. SEPARATION AND PURIFICATION OF GREEN TEA POLYPHENOL COMPONENTS

An example of the procedure for separation and purification of each component of green tea polyphenols is shown in Figure 1. Green tea polyphenols were separated into three fractions with a high porosity polystyrene gel column (particle size, 75-150 µm, Diaion HP-20, Mitsubishi Kagaku Co., Japan; column, 25 ϕ x 1,000 mm) chromatography. A sample of 100 mg green tea polyphenols dissolved in 20 ml water was applied and eluted stepwise with 100 ml of methanol/ H_2O = 1/ 5 (fraction 1 and 2) followed by methanol/ H_2O = 2/ 5 (fraction 3). Elution was performed at a flow rate of 5 ml/min.

Each fraction obtained above was purified with preparative recycling liquid chromatography equipped with GS-310 (particle size, 9 µm; column, 7.6 ϕ x 500 mm; Model LC-908, Japan Analytical Industry Co. Ltd., Japan). The mobile phase consisted of acetonitrile/ H_2O = 3/7, elution was performed at a flow rate of 10 ml/min with monitoring at 280 nm.

The components of the fractions above were analyzed with Waters HPLC Model 600E instrument equipped with Model 717 autosampler and 490E programmable multiwavelength detector (Millipore Co., USA). The column used was Develosil ODS-P-5 (column, 4.6 ϕ x 150 mm; Nomura Chemical Co., Japan). The injection volume was 5 µl, and the mobile phase consisted of acetic acid/acetonitrile/N, N-dimethylformamide/H_2O = 3/1/15/81. The elution was performed at a flow rate of 0.5 ml/ min by monitoring at 280 nm.

The results of HPLC analysis of Fraction 1, 2, and 3 are shown in Figure 2. The elution profile of above Fraction 2 on the recycling liquid chromatography is shown in Figure 3.

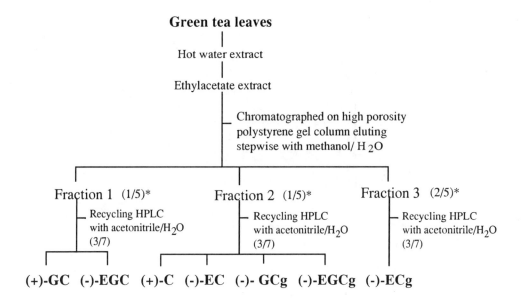

Figure 1. Separation and purification of green tea polyphenols.
*Figure in parenthesese indicates the ratio of methanol to H_2O as the eluent.

III. CHEMICAL AND PHYSICOCHEMICAL PROPERTIES OF GREEN TEA POLYPHENOLS

The data on the chemical and physicochemical properties of green tea polyphenols are summarized based on the reports by various researchers. Figure 4 shows some photochemical properties of the polyphenols together with structures [9-12]. Some data on ^{1}H-NMR, ^{13}C-NMR spectra, hydroxylation pattern, and absolute configuration of several tea polyphenols are shown in Tables 1 [13], 2, and 3 [12], respectively. Also, some chemical reactivities of the polyphenols are given in Table 4 [14].

IV. RECENT DEVELOPMENTS ON CHEMICAL AND PHYSICOCHEMICAL PROPERTIES OF POLYPHENOLS

A. NEW POLYPHENOLS ISOLATED FROM GREEN TEA LEAVES

Four dimeric proanthocyanin gallates, and two novel dimeric flavan-3-ol gallates linked at the B-ring, named theasinensins A and B, together with (-)-epigallocatechin p-coumaroate and (-)-epigallocatechin digallate were isolated, and the structures were established by Nonaka and his colleagues [14]. (-)-epicatechin-3-(3"-O-methylgallate) and (-)-epigallocatechin-3-(3"-O-methylgallate) were isolated and determined by Saijo [15]. The structure and photochemical properties of the polyphenols mentioned above are shown in Figure 5.

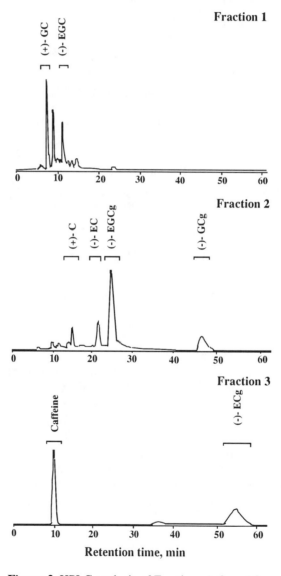

Figure 2. HPLC analysis of Fractions 1, 2, and 3.

Properties of Green Tea Polyphenols 27

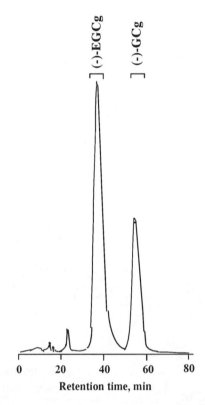

Figure 3. Elution profile of Fraction 2 on the recycling liquid chromatography.

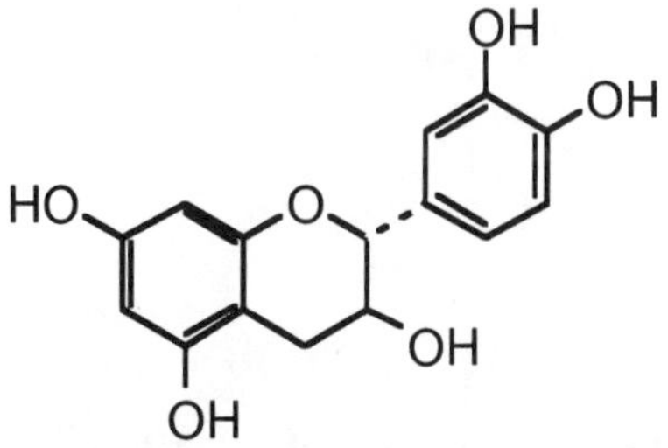

(+)-**Catechin** ((+)-**C**),
$C_{15}H_{14}O_6$, mol wt 290.
m. p. 176°C,
$[\alpha]_D + 18°$,
[9].

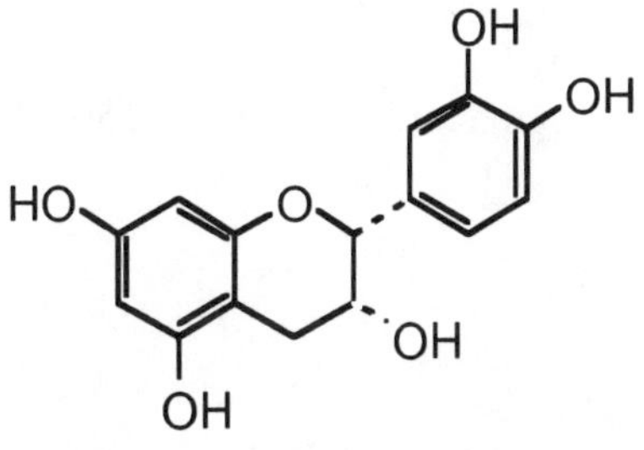

(-)-**Epicatechin** ((-)-**EC**),
$C_{15}H_{14}O_6$, mol wt 290.
m. p. 242°C,
$[\alpha]_D -69°$,
[10].
λ max 280, ε max 3,300,
[11].

Figure 4. Structure, molecular formula, molecular weight, melting point, optical rotation, and maximum absorption wavelength of each component of green tea polyphenols. Reproduced from Hergert and Kurth (1953) [9], Bradfield and Penney (1948) [11], and Birch et al (1957) [12] by permission of the American Chemical Society, Washington D.C.

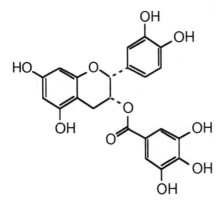

(+)-Gallocatechin((+)-GC),
$C_{15}H_{14}O_7$, mol wt 306.
m. p. 188°C,
$[\alpha]_D$ +15°,
[12].
λ max 271, ε max 1,290,
[11].

(-)-Epigallocatechin ((-)-EGC),
$C_{15}H_{14}O_7$, mol wt 306.
m. p. 218°C,
$[\alpha]_D$ -50°,
[12].

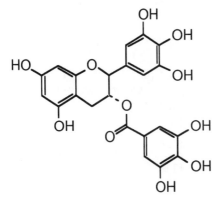

(-)-Epicatechin gallate ((-)-ECg),
$C_{22}H_{18}O_{10}$, mol wt 442.
m. p. 253°C,
$[\alpha]_D$ -177°,
λ max 280, ε max 13,600,
[11].

(-)-Gallocatechin gallate ((-)-GCg),
$C_{22}H_{18}O_{11}$, mol wt 458.
m. p. 216°C,
$[\alpha]_D$ -179°,
λ max 279.5, ε max 9,250, 9,500,
[11].

Figure 4. (Continued).

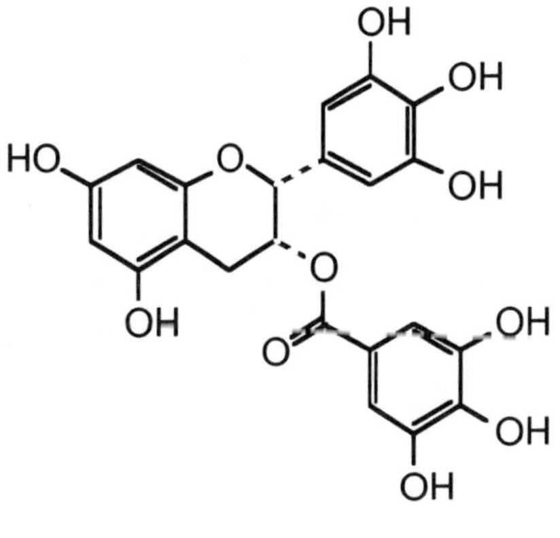

(-)-Epigallocatechin gallate ((-)-EGCg),
$C_{22}H_{18}O_{11}$, mol wt 458.
m. p. 254°C,
$[\alpha]_D$ -190°,
[12].

Figure 4. (Continued).

Table 1
^{1}H- NMR Spectra of Green Tea Polyphenols [1]

	(+)- C	(-)- EC[2]	(+)- GC	(-)- EGC[2]	(-)- ECg[2]	(-)- GCg	(-)- EGCg
C- Ring							
C2- H	4.57 (d, J=8 Hz)	4.88 (s)	4.53 (d, J=8 Hz)	4.81 (s)	5.14 (s)	5.06 (d, J=6 Hz)	4.98 (s)
C3- H	3.97 (m)	4.22 (m)	3.96 (m)	4.18 (m)	5.55 (m)	5.39 (m)	5.53 (m)
C4- H	2.48- 2.88 (m)	2.56- 3.04 (m)	2.47- 2.84 (m)	2.59- 3.00 (m)	2.79- 3.21 (m)	2.73- 2.80 (m)	2.83- 3.32 (m)
A- Ring							
C6- H	5.86 (d, J=2 Hz)	5.92 (d, J=2 Hz)	5.86 (d, J=2 Hz)	5.91 (d, J=2 Hz)	6.06 (s)	5.96 (s)	5.97 (s)
C8- H	5.93 (d, J=2 Hz)	6.02 (d, J=2 Hz)	5.92 (d, J=2 Hz)	6.01 (d, J=2 Hz)	6.06 (s)	5.96 (s)	5.97 (s)
B- Ring							
C2',6'- H			6.40 (s)	6.57 (s)		6.41 (s)	6.52 (s)
C5'- H	6.71- 6.84 (m)	5.96- 7.16 (m)	-	-	6.65- 7.08 (m)	-	-
3- O- Galloyl							
C2", 6"- H	-	-	-	-	7.02 (s)	6.98 (s)	6.96 (s)

[1]The spectral data were recorded on a JEOL GX-400 spectrometer with tetramethylsilane as an internal standard, and chemical shifts were given in δ (ppm). Spectra were run in methanol- d₄ at 400 MHz. s, singlet; d, doublet; m, multiplet.

[2]Reproduced from Nonaka et al. (1983) [13] by permission of the Pharmaceutical Society of Japan, Tokyo.

Table 2
^{13}C- NMR Spectra of Green Tea Polyphenols [1]

	(+)- C	(-)- EC	(+)- GC	(-)- EGC	(-)- ECg	(-)- GCg	(-)- EGCg
C2	82.9	79.9	82.9	79.9	78.7	79.2	77.5
C3	68.8	67.5	68.8	67.5	70.0	71.1	68.8
C4	28.5	29.3	28.1	29.1	26.9	23.7	25.7
C4a	100.9	100.1	100.8	100.1	99.4	99.6	98.3
C6	95.6	95.9	95.6	95.9	95.9	95.6	94.8
C8	96.4	96.5	96.3	96.4	96.6	96.4	95.5
-COO-	-	-	-	-	167.7	167.6	166.6

[1]The spectral data were recorded on a JEOL GX-400 spectrometer with tetramethylsilane as an internal standard, and chemical shifts were given in δ (ppm). Spectra were run in methanol- d_4 at 400 MHz.

Table 3
Hydroxylation Patterns and Absolute Configurations of Special Green Tea Polyphenols [1]

Compounds	Hydroxylation pattern	Absolute configuration
(+)- C	5,7,3',4'	2R:3S
(-)- EC	5,7,3',4'	2R:3R
(+)- GC	5,7,3',4',5'	2R:3S
(-)- EGC	5,7,3',4',5'	2R:3R

[1]Reproduced from Birch et al. (1957) [12] by permission of the Royal Society of Chemistry, Herts.

Table 4

Reactivity of Green Tea Polyphenols with FeCl$_3$, Gelatin, Dilute Sulfuric Acid, and Phloroglucinol

	(-)- EC	(-)- EGC	(-)- ECg	(-)- EGCg
FeCl$_3$	Green	Violet	Blue	Blue
Gelatin	No ppt.	No ppt.	White ppt.	White ppt.
Heating with dilute acid[1]	Reddish brown ppt.	Reddish brown ppt.	Gallic acid and reddish brown ppt.	Gallic acid and reddish brown ppt.
Phloroglucinol reaction	Positive	Positive	Positive	Positive

[1] 5 % sulfuric acid.
Reproduced from Tsujimura and Takasu (1955) [14] by permission of the Japan Society for Bioscience, Biotechnology, and Agrochemistry, Tokyo.

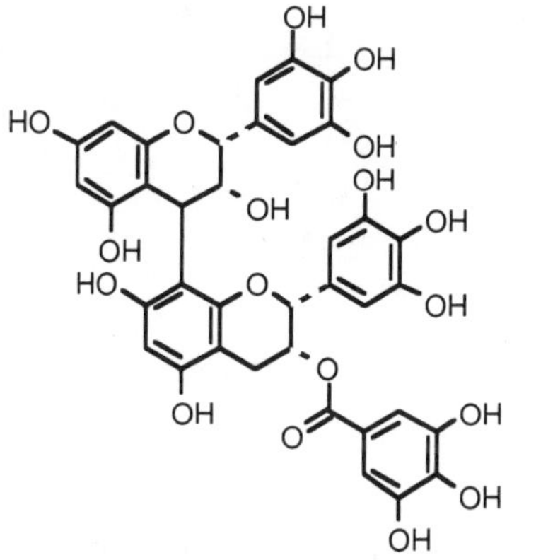

$[\alpha]_D$ -52.7° [13].

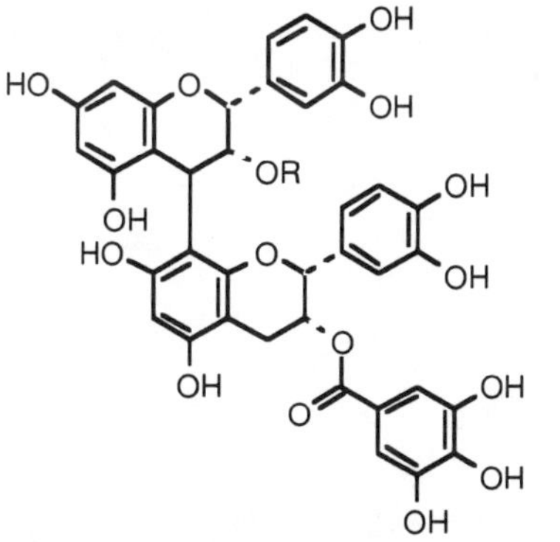

R = H $[\alpha]_D$ -45.8°,
R = G $[\alpha]_D$ -95.2° [13].

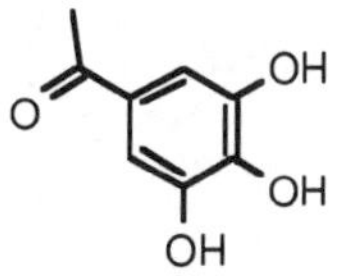

Figure 5. Structures and photochemical properties of several new polyphenols isolated from green tea leaves. Reproduced from Nonaka et al. (1983) [13] by permission of the Pharmaceutical Society of Japan, Tokyo and Saijo (1982) [15] by permission of the Japan Society for Bioscience, Biotechnology, and Agrochemistry, Tokyo.

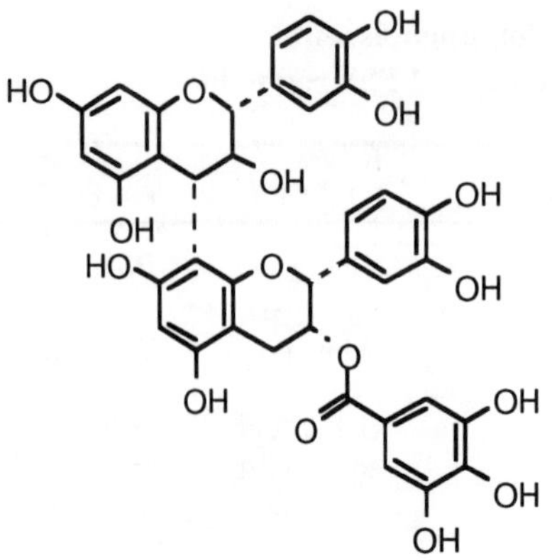

[α]D -255.7° [13].

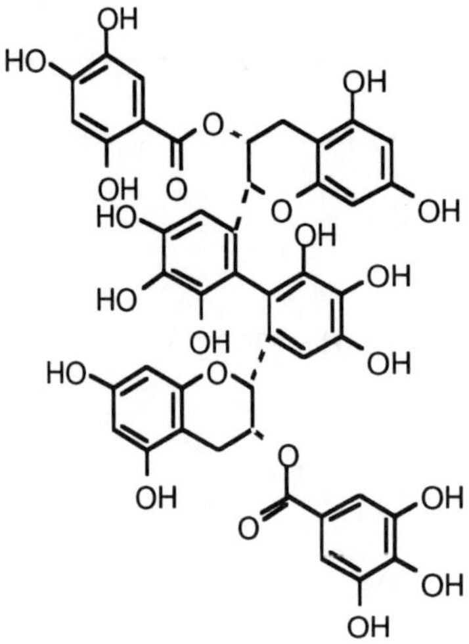

$C_{44}H_{34}O_{22} \cdot 1\,1/2\,H_2O$
[α]D -226.8°,
[θ]20 (mm) -464,000 (220),
0 (239), +40,900 (244),
0 (253), -20,500 (265) [13].

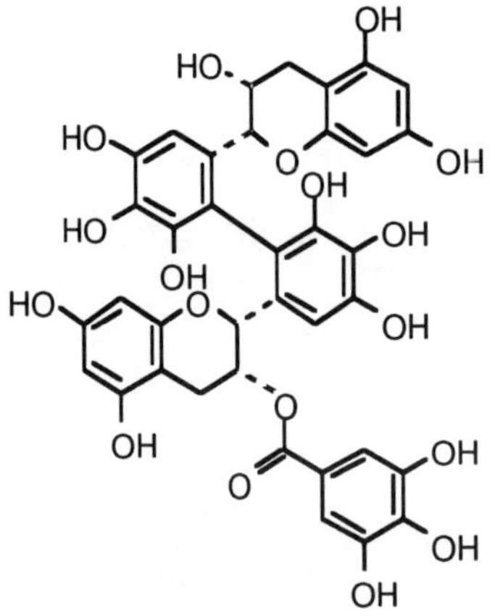

$C_{37}H_{30}O_{18} \cdot 1/2\,H_2O$
[α]D -147.2° [13].

Figure 5. (Continued).

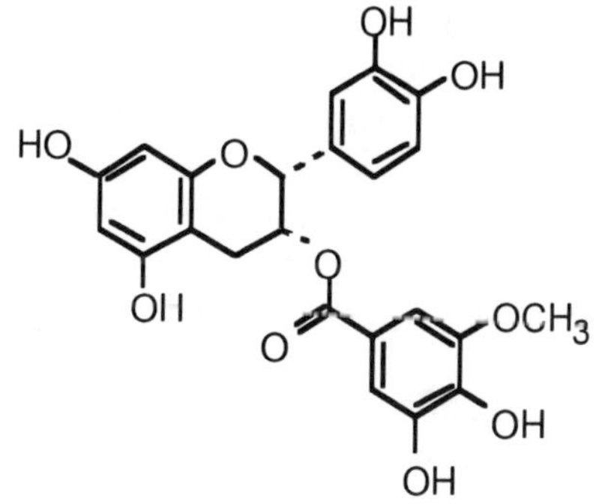

(-)-epicatechin-3-(3"-O-methylgallate)
[α] D -168°,
λ max 280,
IR ν max cm-1: 3,375, 1,685, 1,610, 1,515, 1,460, 1,330, 1,225, 1,140, 1,085 [15].

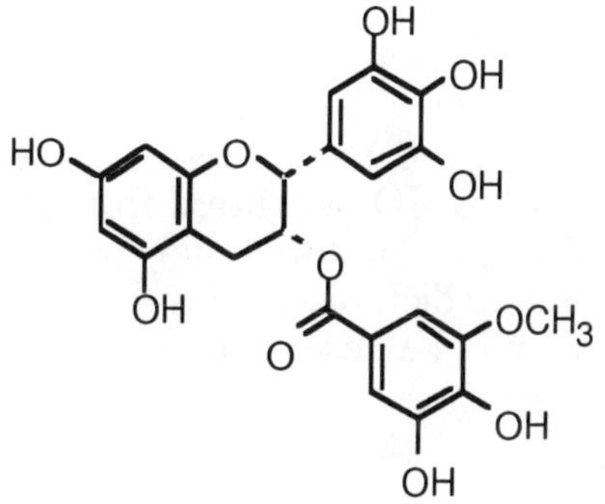

(-)-epigallocatechin-3-(3"-O-methylgallate)
[α] D -162°,
λ max -277,
IR ν max cm-1: 3,375, 1,685, 1,610, 1,515, 1,460, 1,330, 1,225, 1,140, 1,085, 1,015 [15].

Figure 5. (Continued).

B. REACTIVITY OF POLYPHENOLS TO VARIOUS SUBSTANCES

A precipitate formation of (-)-EGCg and (-)-ECg with soybean lipoxygenase (LOX) in the pH range of 4-7 was reported by Sekiya and his colleagues [16], with an accompanying 10-30% loss of the LOX activity. Yeast alcohol dehydrogenase also was precipitated by (-)-EGCg. Polyvinyl pyrrolidone, Tween 20 and Triton X-100 dissociated the LOX from the (-)-EGCg-precipitated LOX. The molecular weight of dissociated LOX (114,000) differed from that of the native LOX (100,000). Enzyme activities of the (-)-EGCg-precipitated LOX and the dissociated LOX from the precipitate were slightly less than that of the native LOX.

Maruyama and his coworkers [6] reported that when the mixture of (-)-EGCg and caffeine with increasing the molar ratio of (-)-EGCg to caffeine from 0:1 to 4:1 was subjected to ^{1}H-NMR measurement (400 MHz), significant up-field shifts were observed in H-8 (Δδ -0.52) and N7-CH$_3$ (Δδ -0.32). The binding or complexing between gallic acid esters and caffeine was reported to be mediated by hydrogen bonding and hydrophobic effects [17]. The binding between gallic acid ester and caffeine was considered to be due to two parallel planer systems of 3.37 Å apart held by reduced hydrophobic interaction with the medium through maximum overlap of the two hydrophobic planes.

The oxidation of (+)-C and (-)-EC in the presence of an excess of cysteine was investigated by Richard and his coworkers [18]. After purification by gel filtration, the structure of the conjugated cysteine was determined by ^{1}H-NMR spectroscopy. Cysteine was attached on the B-ring of (+)-C and (-)-EC. The 2'-position of the B-ring was involved in the formation of the first addition compound, and the 5'-position was in that of the second one. UV Spectra analysis revealed that the conjugation above at the 2'-position and 5'-position occurred at the same rate in equivalent amounts.

The chemical reaction of (-)-EGCg with methyl mercaptan (CH_3SH) was investigated by Yasuda and his colleagues [19]. The reaction product was identified to involve methylthio and/or methylsulfinyl group at 2'- and 5'-positions of the B-ring of (-)-EGCg.

The inclusion complex of (+)-C with cyclodextrins (CDx) was examined by the use of ^{1}H-NMR, UV, and circular dichroism spectroscopies by Smith and his coworkers [20]. The observation of spectral red shift and the presence of isosbestic points in the UV measurements indicated an association between (+)-C and β-CDx. The up-field chemical shifts of (+)-C resonances upon addition of β-CDx were observed in H-6 ($\Delta\delta$ -0.23) and H-8 ($\Delta\delta$ -0.13), and that of β-CDx resonance was observed in H-3" ($\Delta\delta$ -0.159). These findings suggested that the interaction between (+)-C and β-CDx occurred from the side containing secondary hydrogen groups. The apparent formation constant estimated was 8700 M^{-1} in the analysis by the circular dichroism measurements.

Epimerization and oxidation of polyphenols will be described in detail in the following chapter.

REFERENCES

1. **Haslam, E.,** Polyphenols - vegetable tannins, in *Plant Polyphenols*, Cambridge University Press, Cambridge, 1989, p 9.
2. **Ahn, Y.-J., Kawamura, T., Kim, M., Yamamoto, T., and Mitsuoka, T.,** Tea polyphenols: Selective growth inhibitors of *Clostridium* spp., *Agric. Biol. Chem*, **55**, 1425, 1991.
3. **Shi, S. T., Wang, Z.-Y., Smith, T. J., Hong, J.-Y., Chen, W.-F., Ho, C.-T., and Yang, C. S.,** Effects of green tea and black tea on 4-(methylnitrosamino)-1-(3-pyridyl)-1-butanone bioactivation, DNA methylation, and lung tumorigenesis in A/J mice, *Cancer Res.*, **54**, 4641, 1994.
4. **Mukhtar, H., Katiyar, S. K., and Agarwal, R.,** Green tea and skin-anticarcinogenic effects, *J. Invest. Dermatol.*, **102**, 3, 1994.
5. **Cai, Y., Gaffney, S. H., Lilley, T. H., Magnolato, D., Martin, R., Spencer, C. M., and Haslam, E.,** Polyphenol interactions. Part 4. Model studies with caffeine and cyclodextrins, *J. Chem. Soc. Perkin Trans.*, **2**, 2197, 1990.
6. **Maruyama, N., Suzuki, Y., Sakata, K., Yagi, A., and Ina, K.,** *Proceedings of the International Symposium on Tea Science,* Kurofune Printing Co. Ltd., Shizuoka, 1991, p 145.
7. **Murray, N., Williamson, M. P., Lilley, T. H., and Haslam, E.,** Studies of the interaction between salivary proline-rich proteins and a polyphenol by ^{1}H-NMR spectroscopy, *Eur. J. Biochem.*, **219**, 923, 1994.

8. **Bingying, G. and Qikun, C.,** Reaction of tea infusion components with metal ions and its application to preparation of pure polyphenols, in *Proceedings of the International Symposium on Tea Science,* Kurofune Printing Co. Ltd., Shizuoka, 1991, p 86.
9. **Hergert, H. L. and Kurth, E. T.,** The isolation and properties of catechol from white fir bark, *J. Org. Chem.*, 521, 1953.
10. **Biggs, R. P., Cooper, W. L., Hazleton, E. O., Nierenstein, M., and Price, P. H.,** Stereoisomeric catechins, *J. Am. Chem. Soc.*, 53, 1500, 1931.
11. **Bradfield, A. E. and Penney, M.,** The catechins of green tea. Part 2, *J. Chem. Soc.*, 2249, 1948.
12. **Birch, A. J., Clark-Lewis, J. W., and Robertson, A. V.,** The relative and absolute configurations of catechins and epicatechins, *J. Chem. Soc.*, 3586, 1957.
13. **Nonaka, G., Kawahara, O., and Nishioka, I.,** Tannins and related compounds. XV. A new class of dimeric flavan-3-ol gallates, theasinensins A and B, and proanthocyanidin gallates from green tea leaf. (1), *Chem. Pharm. Bull.*, 31, 3906, 1983.
14. **Tsujimura, M. and Takasu, E.,** On the tea tannins in green tea. Isolation of tea tannin 2 in crystalline state, *Nippon Nougeikagaku Kaishi (in Japanese)*, 29, 407, 1955.
15. **Saijo, R.,** Isolation and chemical structures of two new catechins from fresh tea leaf, *Agric. Biol. Chem.*, 46, 1969, 1982.
16. **Sekiya, J., Kajiwara, T., Monma, T., and Hatanaka, A.,** Interaction of tea catechins with proteins: Formation of protein precipitate, *Agric. Biol. Chem.*, 48, 1963, 1984.
17. **Martin, R., Lilley, T. H., Bailey, N. A., Falshaw, C. P., Haslam, E., Magnolato, D., and Begley, N. J.,** Polyphenol-caffeine complexation, *J. Chem. Soc. Chem. Commun.*, 105, 1986.
18. **Richard, F. C., Goupy, P. M., Nicolas, J. J., Lacombe, J.-M., and Pavia, A. A.,** Cysteine as an inhibitor of enzymatic browning. 1. Isolation and characterization of addition compounds formed during oxidation of phenolics by apple polyphenol oxidase, *J. Agric. Food Chem.*, 39, 841, 1991.
19. **Yasuda, H. and Arakawa, T.,** Deodorizing mechanism of (-)-epigallocatechin gallate against methyl mercaptan, *Biosci. Biotech. Biochem.*, 59, 1232, 1995.
20. **Smith, V. K., Ndou, T. T., and Warner, I. M.,** Spectroscopic study of the interaction of catechin with α-, β-, and γ-cyclodextrins, *J. Phys. Chem.*, 98, 8627, 1994.

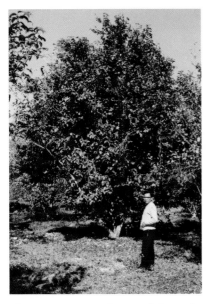

Plate 1. A matured tree of *Camellia sinensis* var. *assamica* (about 40 years old) at Gillapukhri Tea Estate, Assam, India. (Courtesy of Professor M. Hashimoto, Meijo University, Nagoya, Japan.)

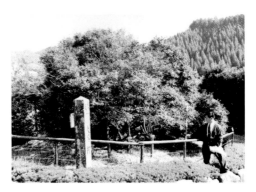

Plate 2. Matured trees of *Camellia sinensis* var. *sinensis* (about 330 years old) at Ureshino-cho, Saga Prefecture, Japan. (Courtesy of the Education Committee in Ureshino-cho, Saga Prefecture, Japan.)

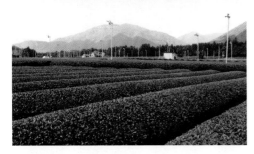

Plate 3. A typical tea plantation in Japan.

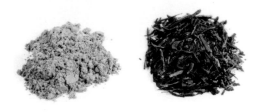

Plate 4. Appearance of Matcha (left) and Sencha (right).

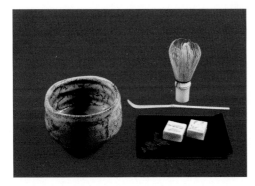

Plate 5. Tools for the traditional manner of drinking Matcha.

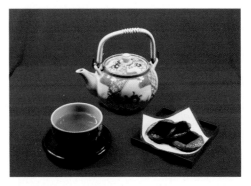

Plate 6. Sencha is one of the most popular beverages in Japan.

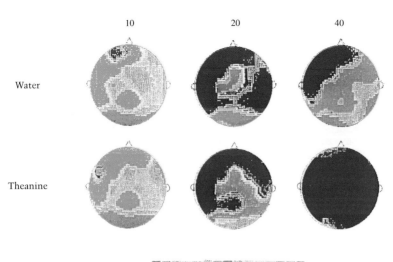

Plate 7. Changes in appearance of the α-brain wave. Differences in appearance and strength of the α-wave become clearer 40 min. after the intake of a theanine solution (200 mg/100 ml water).

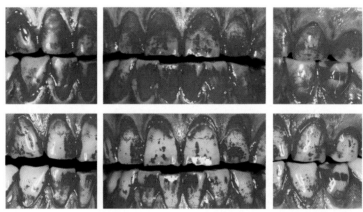

Plate 8. Teeth of subjects rinsed without (top) and with 0.05% tea polyphenols (bottom).

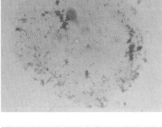

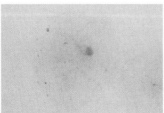

Plate 9. Adherence of bacterial cells onto human buccal epithelial cells without (top) and with 125 μg/ml green tea polyphenols (bottom).

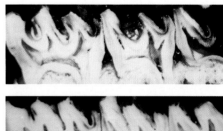

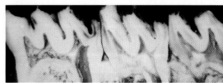

Plate 10. Sections of fuchsin-stained teeth of rats fed on a control diet (top) and a diet containing 0.1% green tea polyphenols (bottom).

Chapter 4

ANTIOXIDATIVE ACTIVITY OF TEA POLYPHENOLS

M. Koketsu

TABLE OF CONTENTS

I. Introduction
II. Antioxidative Activity of Tea Polyphenols on Fats and Oils
III. Antidiscoloring Effect of Green Tea Polyphenols
IV. Antioxidative Activity of Individual Catechins
V. Oxidative Products of Catechins and the Mechanism of Antioxidative Action
VI. Effect of Tea Extract *In Vitro* and *In Vivo* as an Antioxidant
References

I. INTRODUCTION

Many papers have been published so far on the physiological and pharmacological functions of green tea. The effective principles of green tea "polyphenols," are chemically interesting since they are considered to be a radical scavenger and have now attracted many researchers' attention.

The antioxidative activity of green tea was found to be due to the several polyphenols it contains [1-6]. Tea polyphenols are widely used as a natural antioxidant for the prevention of oxidation of edible oils or discoloring of reddish foods in color. Also, the tea polyphenols were found to show several biochemical activities such as inhibition of bacterial mutation [7], inhibition of HIV reverse transcriptase activity [8], anticaries effects [9-11], antiviral activity, or preventive effect from cancer [12-14], as are mentioned in other chapters of this book. The antioxidative activity of the polyphenols shown against fats and oils and some colored foods are described in this chapter. The mechanism of antioxidative action of polyphenols and antioxidative effect *in vitro* and *in vivo* of polyphenols are also mentioned.

II. ANTIOXIDATIVE ACTIVITY OF TEA POLYPHENOLS ON FATS AND OILS

Edible fats and oils are susceptible to rancidity, and in their utilization in food manufacturing, antioxidants are usually added. We examined the antioxidative activity using an alcohol solution of tea polyphenols. The rancidity of lard oil was monitored by measuring the increase of peroxide value (PV), according to the autoxidative method [15]. Tea polyphenols clearly showed a suppressive effect on oxidation of oil, and the effect was concentration-dependent. The antioxidative effect of tea polyphenols was more effective as compared to tocopherol, as shown in Figure 1. It is interesting that unlike tea polyphenols, tocopherol did not show concentration-dependence, and the addition of more than 400 ppm of tocopherol did not produce any antioxidative effect under these conditions.

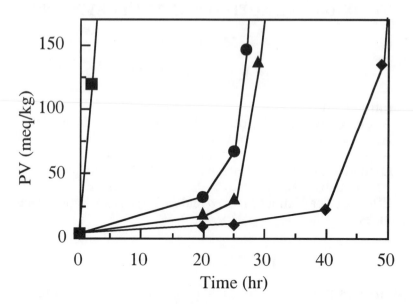

Figure 1. Antioxidative activity of tea polyphenols on lard oil. 400 ppm of natural tocopherol and 400 or 600 ppm of tea polyphenols were added to lard oil, respectively. –■–, control; –●–, 400 ppm natural tocopherol; –▲–, 400 ppm tea polyphenols; –◆–, 600 ppm tea polyphenols.

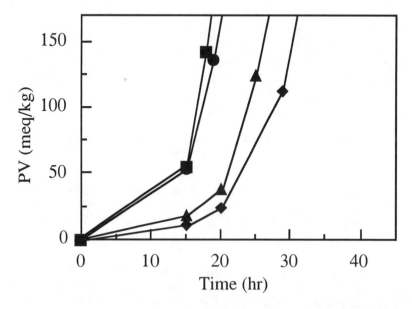

Figure 2. Antioxidative activity of tea polyphenols against soybean oil. 400 ppm of natural tocopherol and 400 or 600 ppm of tea polyphenols were added to soybean oil, respectively. –■–, control; –●–, 400 ppm natural tocopherol; –▲–, 400 ppm tea polyphenol –◆–, 600 ppm tea polyphenols.

The inhibitory effect of tea polyphenols on rancid formation of soybean oil was also examined under the same condition as lard. The fact was interesting that tocopherol showed no effect for depressing rancid formation of soybean oil while tea polyphenols were distinctly effective and suppressed the oxidation of the oil. This effect of polyphenols was also concentration-dependent (Figure 2).

The antioxidative effect of tea polyphenols against dough noodle was also examined. Frying of the dough noodle was done at 120°C for 5 min with lard oil with or without antioxidant, and the fried noodles were kept at 37°C in an incubator. To estimate PV, the noodles were extracted with a mixture of chloroform and methanol (2:1; v/v), the extract was concentrated in vacuo, and the residual oil was subjected to estimation of PV. The tea polyphenols showed a strong antioxidative activity as compared to the control. The addition of green tea polyphenols in the lard oil improved the oxidative stability of fried noodle (Figure 3). This stabilizing effect of tea polyphenols was also dependent on the concentration.

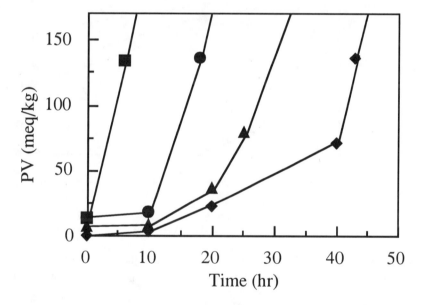

Figure 3. Antioxidative activity of tea polyphenols against lard oil in fried noodles. 400 ppm of natural tocopherol and 400 or 600 ppm of tea polyphenols were added, respectively, to lard oil mixed into noodle dough to be fried.–■–, control; –●–, 400 ppm natural tocopherol; –▲–, 400 ppm tea polyphenols; –◆–, 600 ppm tea polyphenols.

III. ANTIDISCOLORING EFFECT OF GREEN TEA POLYPHENOLS

Red coloring is widely used in various foods industries as well as confectioneries. Also, some foods or fishes are naturally red colored and in numerous cases, the natural reddish color is due to carotenoids. Carotenoids have many double bonds in their molecules and are highly oxidizable. The oxidation of carotenoids is initiated by ultraviolet rays, etc., and finally the structure breaks down and loses the color.

The antidiscoloring effect of tea polyphenols was examined using beverages, margarine, and red-colored fish as samples. The beverages employed were prepared as a model by mixing the following ingredients: water-soluble β-carotene (0.04%), ethanol (2%), sugar syrup (20.0%), citric acid (1.0%), water (77%), and antioxidant (0-0.1%). The prepared beverages were kept at room temperature, and the β-carotene content was periodically measured at 466 nm with a spectrophotometer. The beverage without the antioxidant was discolored within 10 days while the beverage with tea polyphenols maintained the color for more than 40 days. The results are shown in Figure 4, indicating that the antidiscoloring effect of tea polyphenols was greater than L-ascorbate.

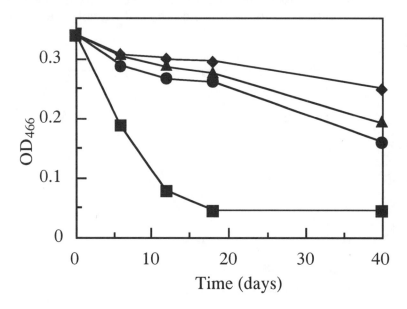

Figure 4. Antidiscoloring effect of tea polyphenols against β-carotene in beverages. –■–, control; –●–, 0.05 % L-ascorbate; –▲–, 0.05 % tea polyphenols; –◆–, 0.10 % tea polyphenols.

The antidiscoloring effect of tea polyphenols for margarine was also examined. The margarine samples with or without tea polyphenols were exposed to UV radiation set up at 254 nm and evaluated by estimating the superficial white and yellow color density as an index of oxidation (Color ace model TC-1, Tokyo Denshoku Co., Ltd., Japan). The margarine mixed with tea polyphenols was found to retain the yellow color, indicating efficiency of tea polyphenols against discoloring by UV rays, as shown in Figure 5. This effect was confirmed in other experiments using several reddish-colored fish containing carotenoids such as salmon, trout, etc. (Table 1) [16]. Carotenoids in the samples were discolored as the time passed after death of the fish. Tea polyphenols were also found to be effective in suppressing the discoloration of fish meat.

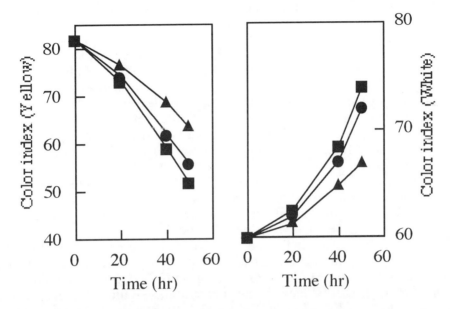

Figure 5. Antidiscoloring effect of tea polyphenols against β-carotene in margarine. —■—, control; —●—, 50 ppm tea polyphenols; —▲—, 400 ppm tea polyphenols.

Table 1
Distributuion of Carotenoids in Several Salmon Species

	Red salmon	Silver salmon	Brown trout
β-Carotene	0.5	2.7	1.6
Echinenone	0.6	1.8	–
Cryptoxanthin	0.7	0.7	1.6
Canthaxanthin	0.4	–	0.9
Tunaxanthin	–	4.7	–
Lutein	trace	1.1	9.0
Antheraxanthin	9.3	13.8	–
Zeaxanthin	6.1	24.6	24.5
Salmoxanthin	28.9	15.7	trace
Diadinoxanthin	–	–	11.9
Unidentified	16.6	3.6	10.5
Triol	3.0	8.1	–
Tetrol	15.6	11.5	0.2
Astacene	6.5	10.1	0.5
β-Doradecin	1.3	1.9	–

Reproduced from Matsuno (1978) [16] by permission of Nippon Suisan Gakkai, Tokyo.

IV. ANTIOXIDATIVE ACTIVITY OF INDIVIDUAL CATECHINS

The antioxidative effect of several kinds of tea extracts was investigated using canola oil [17]. The ethanol extract of green tea showed a strong antioxidative activity on canola oil compared with butylated hydroxytoluene (BHT). In contrast, the extract of oolong tea, which is a semi-fermented product, exhibited only a moderate antioxidative activity. The extract of black tea, which is a completely fermented product, showed little or no protective effect against canola oil. Since tea polyphenols are destroyed partly or completely during the fermentation for manufacturing of oolong or black tea, it may be reasonable that antioxidative activity of oolong and black tea is weaker than green tea.

The degree of antioxidative activity of individual catechins was examined by several antioxidative assay systems. The antioxidative activities of polyphenols were in the following order: (-)-epicatechin-3-gallate (ECg) > (-)-epicatechin (EC), (-)-epigallocatechin-3-gallate (EGCg) > (-)-epigallocatechin (EGC) in the β-carotene-linoleate model system [18]. On the other hand, the antioxidative activities of polyphenols on soybean oil or lard oil were in the order: EGCg > EGC > ECg > EC [3, 5, 6]. The 1,1-diphenyl-2-picrylhydrazyl (DPPH) radical-scavenging ability of the catechins was EGCg > ECg > EGC > EC. EGCg, ECg, EGC, theaflavin digallate, theaflavin monogallate, and theaflavin showed higher DPPH radical- and superoxide-scavenging abilities than BHT [19]. Although there is little difference in various assay systems examined, EGCg, which is the major component among tea polyphenols, shows the strongest antioxidative activity. The antioxidative activity of catechins was proportional to the number of hydrogen radical donors of catechins. Tea catechins showed a synergistic effect with caffeine [3], malic acid, tartaric acid, and citric acid, especially with, tocopherol and L-ascorbic acid [6]. Tocopherol, which is widely used as a natural antioxidant of lipids, is greatly effective for stabilization of lipids when applied together with catechins. The synergistic effect shown by mixing tocopherol and catechins suggests that tocopherol is prevented from oxidative destruction by the oxide radical-scavenging activity of catechins [20].

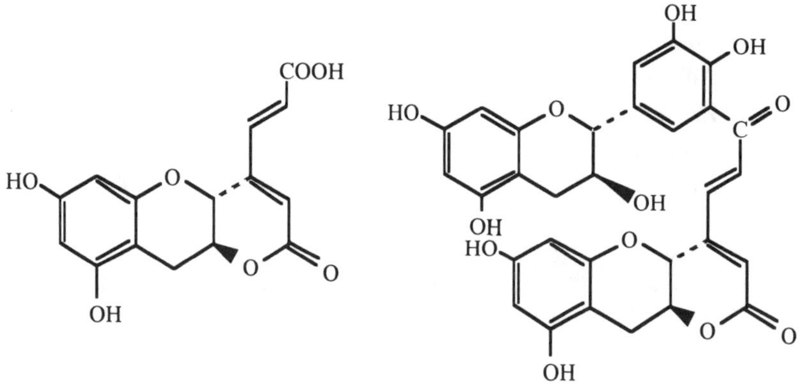

Figure 6. Oxidized products of (+)-catechin.

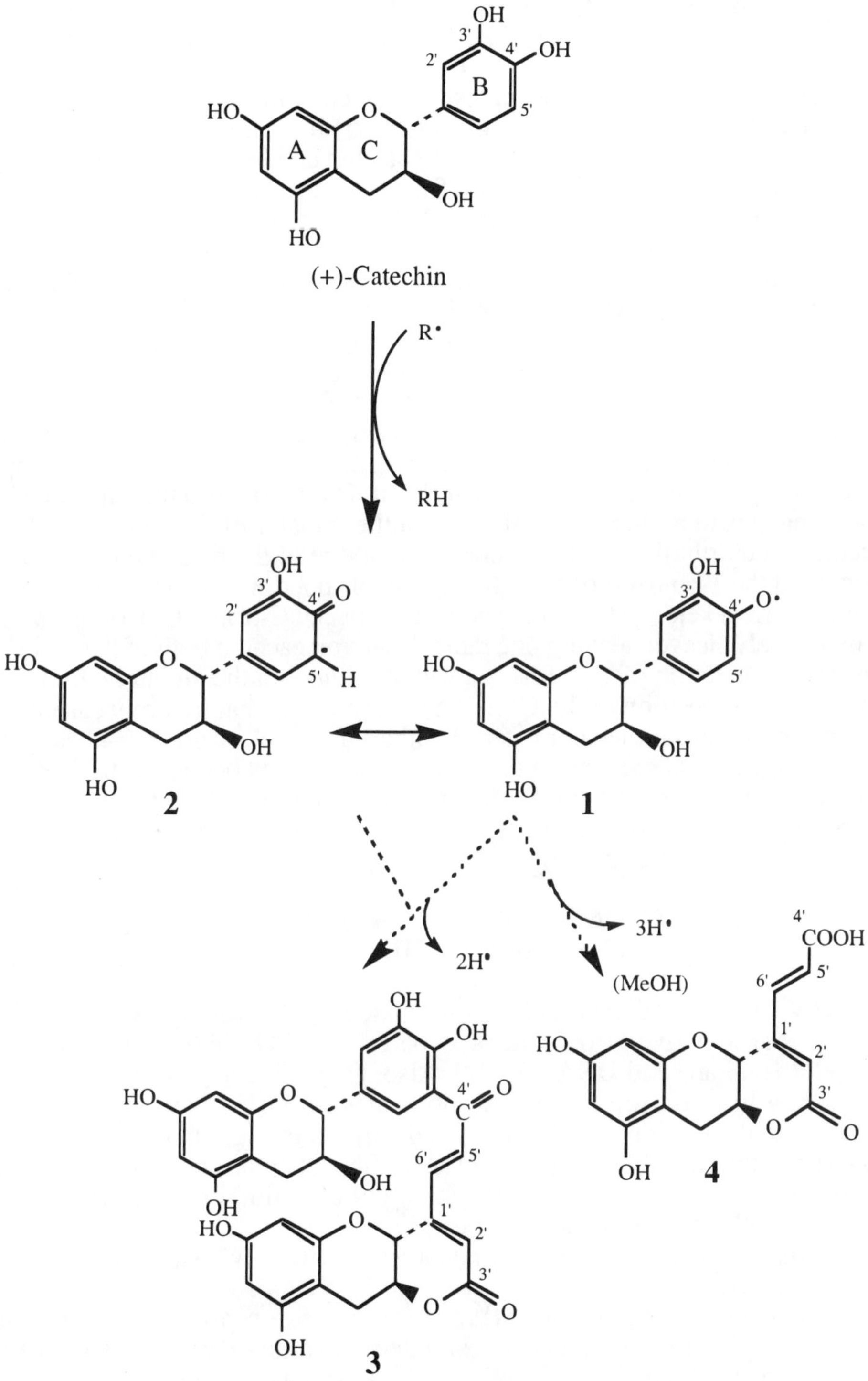

Figure 7. Proposed mechanism of formation of oxidation products of (+)-catechin. Reproduced from Nakayama and Hirose (1994) [25] by permission of F F I Journal, Osaka.

V. OXIDATIVE PRODUCTS OF CATECHINS AND THE MECHANISM OF ANTIOXIDATIVE ACTION

In order to postulate the mechanism involved in the antioxidative action of catechins, Hirose and her colleagues [21-25] investigated the structure of oxidized products of the mixture of (+)-catechin and methyl ester of fatty acid that was subjected to irradiation with fluorescence, and the products shown in Figure 6 were observed to be formed during the radical-scavenging reaction that prevents the lipid peroxidation.

The formation of oxidation products was also confirmed when ethyl acetate solution of (+)-catechin was irradiated under a fluorescent lamp in the presence of 2,2'-azobis [2-methylpropanenitrile] as a radical initiator. On the basis of these products, Hirose and her colleagues speculate the mechanism of radical scavenging action of (+)-catechin as shown in Figure 7 [25].

(+)-Catechin liberates the hydrogen radical from hydroxy groups of 3'- and 4'-positions in B ring, and the hydrogen radical joins other radicals, e.g., lipid peroxide by which this radical is stabilized. On the other hand, the catechin itself changes to a phenoxy radical, then the transfer of the radical electron occurs by contribution of the resonance structure of the benzene ring and the carbons at the 3'- and 4'-positions form a double bond with a remaining oxygen atom to form a ketone structure. The bond between C-3' and C-4' of the B ring is oxidatively cleaved leaving one radical electron each on both of the carbons. The radical electron of C-3' forms a lactone ring with the alcoholic hydroxyl group of the 3-position of the C ring in the same way that hydroxy carboxylic acid forms an intramolecular ester. Another radical electron of C-4' captures the hydroxy radical existing in the reaction system and becomes stable by the formation of carboxylic acid. By this reaction process, catechin can scavenge four radicals per mole, and the idea above may explain the mechanism of the antioxidative action of catechin.

VI. EFFECT OF TEA EXTRACT *IN VITRO* AND *IN VIVO* AS AN ANTIOXIDANT

Active oxygen radicals such as superoxide (O^{2-}), hydroxy radical (HO·), and the radical derived from hydrogen peroxide (H_2O_2) deterioratively affect the cell membrane and DNA [26, 27]. Also, they are known to be involved in aging and in initiation and promotion of tumors (Figure 8). In order to antagonize the influence of the toxic radical, living organisms are bestowed with superoxide dismutase (SOD) and also with glutathione peroxidase, vitamin E, and several other antioxidants which act to maintain a certain balance between oxidation and reduction potentials.

Tea polyphenols also show antioxidative activity *in vivo* as well as *in vitro* and can prevent living cells from oxidative impairment. Terao and his coworkers [28] prepared large unilamellar liposomes composed of egg yolk phosphatidylcholine (PC) and investigated the antioxidative effects of EC, ECg, and quercetin on lipid peroxidation exposing the suspension to a water-soluble radical initiator, 2,2'-azobis (2-aminopropane) hydrochloride (AAPH). The inhibitory effects of those flavonoids lasted longer than that of α-tocopherol. EC and ECg were located near the surface of the biomembrane much like phospholipid bilayers fit for scavenging aqueous oxygen radical. Namiki and Osawa [29] have investigated the effect of polyphenols as antioxidants on the formation of an oxygen radical. Rabbit blood cells were subjected to autoxidation with or without antioxidant, and the peroxide generated was measured. These peroxide formation under these conditions was compared with that of the control, expressing the degree of antioxidation effect. Among the tea polyphenols, EGCg exhibited the strongest antioxidative activity, and ECg was next. The activity of the two compounds was superior to α-tocopherol (Figure 9).

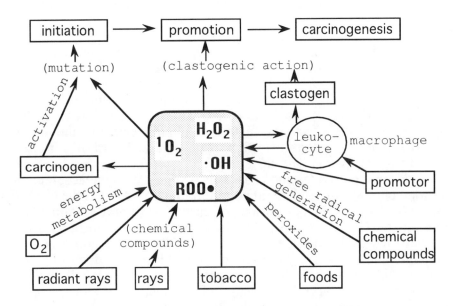

Figure 8. The relationships between carcinogenesis and the active oxygens.

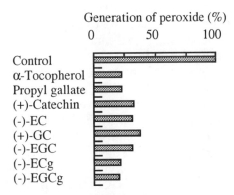

Figure 9. Antioxidative activity of polyphenols shown by the rabbit blood cells assay system. Reproduced from Namiki and Osawa (1986) [29] by permission of Plenum Publishing Co., New York.

The low density lipoprotein (LDL), which is the major carrier of blood cholesterol, is known as the principal lipoprotein susceptible to oxidative modification, and thus the antioxidative activities of natural antioxidants were investigated by several researchers against LDL in the presence of Cu^{2+} to mediate the oxidation. The capacity to prolong the lag-time before the onset of the conjugated diene formation was: sesaminol > quercetin > EGCg > theaflavin myricetin > BHT > α-tocopherol. The effect of EGCg on cholesteryl ester degradation and on apolipoprotein B 100 fragmentation in the Cu^{2+}-mediated oxidative modification of LDL was far superior to BHT and α-tocopherol [30, 31]. Sano and his colleagues [32] investigated the antioxidative effects in the liver and kidney of rats fed on diets containing 3% green tea or black tea powder. The test was carried out by the tissue slice-antioxidant assay system. After 50 days feeding on the diets, the liver slices obtained from the green and black tea-supplemented rats showed significant inhibitory effects against *tert*-butyl hydroperoxide-induced lipid peroxidation. As for the kidney, the antioxidant effect was observed only in the green tea-fed rats. These results demonstrated that dietary green and black tea show antioxidant effects on tissue lipid peroxidation. Kimura and his colleagues [33] investigated the effect of tea extracts on lipid metabolic injury in rats fed peroxidized oil. Oral administration of peroxidized corn oil for one week induced a hyperlipemia with the elevation of serum triglycerides, free fatty acids, and lipid peroxides and caused liver injury with the accumulation of liver total cholesterol, triglycerides, and lipid peroxides and the elevation of serum glutamic oxaloacetic transaminase (GOT) and glutamic pyruvic transaminase (GPT) as compared to the control rats. The green tea-fed group showed better results than the black tea- or oolong tea-fed group against lipid metabolic injury. The green tea-fed group had less elevation of blood GPT, free fatty acids from neutral lipid and lipid peroxides, and also slightly reduced elevation of liver triglycerides. Oolong and black tea did not show antioxidative effects like green tea. In a similar test, the *in vivo* antioxidative activities of tea catechins were examined. The effects of dietary tea catechins on the levels of α-tocopherol and lipid peroxidation in both plasma and erythrocytes were examined in rats fed on high palm and perilla oil diets. The addition of tea catechins to these diets significantly prevented the α-tocopherol concentration from decreasing and slightly reduced the lipid peroxidation in the plasma. Tea catechins are likely to act as an antioxidant *in vivo* [34]. These results indicate that green tea extracts have the ability to suppress the formation of lipid peroxide *in vivo* in which the experimental animals are subjected to excessive intake of peroxidized oil or unsaturated fatty acid.

The relationship between antioxidative activity, antimutagenicity, and oxidative DNA damage has been reported. The antioxidative activity of tea extracts has been observed to correlate well with the antimutagenicity [35]. The oxidative DNA damage, mediated by active oxygen radical, is known to induce carcinogenesis [36]. 8-Hydroxydeoxyguanosine (8-OHdG) is known as a reliable marker for oxidative DNA damage *in vivo* [37, 38] and *in vitro* [39]. Also, it is now clear that several carcinogens specifically induce 8-OHdG formation in their target organs. Green tea or EGCg inhibited the formation of 8-OHdG in lung as well as pulmonary tumorigenesis in mice [40-43]. Wei and Frenkel [44] reported that green tea suppresses the carcinogenesis-promoting activity of 12-O-tetradecanoyl-phorbol-13-acetate in SENCAR mice, accompanied by a decrease in 8-OHdG formation. Hasegawa and his coworkers [45] reported that green tea solution reduced hepatic lipid peroxide levels and effectively blocked oxidative DNA damage in liver as well as hepatotoxicity of rats treated with 2-nitropropane as a hepatocarcinogen. Inagake and his colleagues [46] reported that drinking green tea extract for 10 days prior to a 1,2-dimethylhydrazine injection, which is carcinogenic to rat and liver, significantly inhibited the formation of 8-OHdG in the colon showing that the green tea extract protects colonic mucosa from oxidative damage.

As mentioned above, green tea extracts or tea polyphenols show antioxidative effects both *in vitro* and *in vivo* and seem to be promising compounds in the prevention of several diseases by their antioxidative function.

REFERENCES

1. **Kajimoto, G.**, On the antioxidative components and antiseptic components in tea. Part I. Antioxidant action and antiseptic action of materials extracted with alcohol and water from tea, *Nihon Shokuhin Kogyo Gakkaishi (in Japanese)*, **10**, 1, 1963.
2. **Kajimoto, G., Ikeda, Y., and Mukai, K.**, On the antioxidative components and antiseptic components in tea. Part IV. Antioxidative actions of materials extracted with various organic solvent from tea-grounds, *Eiyo to Shokuryo (in Japanese)*, **22**, 473, 1969.
3. **Kajimoto, G.**, On the antioxidative components and antiseptic components in tea. Part III. The synergistic action of caffeine to catechin components, *Nihon Shokuhin Kogyo Gakkaishi (in Japanese)*, **10**, 365, 1963.
4. **Kajimoto, G.**, On the antioxidative components and antiseptic components in tea. Part II. Reference of antioxidative components and antiseptic components contained in tea by paper chromatography, *Nihon Shokuhin Kogyo Gakkaishi (in Japanese)*, **10**, 3, 1963.
5. **Lea, C. H. and Swoboda, A. T.**, The antioxidant action of some polyphenolic constituents of tea, *Chem. & Ind.*, 1073, 1957.
6. **Matsuzaki, T. and Hara, Y.**, Antioxidative activity of tea leaf catechins, *Nippon Nogeikagaku Kaishi (in Japanese)*, **59**, 129, 1985.
7. **Kada, T., Kaneko, K., Matsuzaki, S., and Matsuzaki, T.**, Detection and chemical identification of natural biomutagens: a case of green tea factor, *Mutation Res.*, **150**, 269, 1985.
8. **Nakane, H. and Ono, K.**, Differential inhibitory effects of some catechins derivatives on the activities of HIV reverse transcriptase and cellular deoxyribonucleic acid and RNA polymerase, *Biochemistry*, **28**, 2841, 1990.
9. **Sakanaka, S., Kim, M., Taniguchi, M., and Yamamoto, T.**, Antibacterial substances in Japanese green tea extract against *Streptococcus mutans*, a cariogenic bacterium, *Agric. Biol. Chem.*, **53**, 2307, 1989.
10. **Sakanaka, S., Shimura, N., Aizawa, M., Kim, M., and Yamamoto, T.**, Preventive effect of green tea polyphenols against dental caries in conventional rats, *Biosci. Biotech. Biochem.*, **56**, 592, 1992.

11. **Sakanaka, S., Sato, T., Kim, M., and Yamamoto, T.,** Inhibitory effects of green tea polyphenols on glucan synthesis and cellular adherence of cariogenic streptococci, *Agric. Biol. Chem.*, **54**, 2925, 1990.
12. **Hirose, M., Hoshiya, T., Akagi, K., Futakuchi, M., and Ito, N.,** Inhibition of mammary gland carcinogenesis by green tea catechins and other naturally occurring antioxidants in female Sprague-Dawley rats pretreated with 7,12-dimethylbenz[*a*]anthracene, *Cancer Lett.*, **83**, 149, 1994.
13. **Hirose, M., Akagi, K., Hasegawa, R., Yaono, M., Satoh, T., Hara, Y., Wakabayashi, K., and Ito, N.,** Chemoprevention of 2-amino-1-methyl-6-phenylimidazo[4,5-b]-pyridine (PhIP)-induced mammary gland carcinogenesis by antioxidants in F344 female rats, *Carcinogenesis*, **16**, 217, 1995.
14. **Zhi, Y. W., Mou-Tuan, H., You-Rong, L., Xie, J.-G., Kenneth, R. R., Harold, L. N., Chi-Tang, H., Chung, S. Y., and Conney, A. H.,** Inhibitory effects of black tea, green tea, decaffeinated black tea, and decaffeinated green tea on ultraviolet B light-induced skin carcinogenesis in 7,12-dimethybenz[*a*]anthracene-initiated SKH-1 mice, *Cancer Res.*, **54**, 3428, 1994.
15. **Buege, J. A. and Aust, S. D.,** POV measurement, *Meth. Enzymol.*, **52**, 302, 1978.
16. **Matsuno, T.,** The distribution of carotenoids in marine animals, in *Carotenoids of marine animals (in Japanese)*, The Japanese Society of Fisheries Science, Ed., Koseisha Koseikaku Co., Ltd., Tokyo, 1978, p 23.
17. **Chen, Z. Y., Chan, P. T., Ma, H. M., Fung, K. P., and Wang, J.,** Antioxidative effect of ethanol tea extracts on oxidation of canola oil, *J. Am. Oil Chem. Soc.*, **73**, 375, 1996.
18. **Amarowicz, R. and Shahidi, F.,** Antioxidant activity of green tea catechins in β-carotene-linoleate model system, *J. Food Lipids*, **2**, 47, 1995.
19. **Chen, C.-W. and Ho, C.-T.,** Antioxidant properties of polyphenols extracted from green and black teas, *J. Food Lipids*, **2**, 35, 1995.
20. **Kajimoto, G., Okajima, N., Takaoka, M., Yoshida, H., and Shibahara, A.,** Effects of catechins on thermal decomposition of tocopherol in heated oils, *Nippon Eiyo Shokuryo Gakkaishi (in Japanese)*, **41**, 213, 1988.
21. **Hirose, Y., Fujita, T., Shima, S., and Nakayama, M.,** An oxidative dimeric product of (+)-catechin by radical reaction in the dark, *J. Jpn. Oil Chem. Soc.*, **44**, 491, 1995.
22. **Hirose, Y., Yamaoka, H., and Nakayama, M.,** Oxidation product of (+)-catechin from lipid peroxidation, *Agric. Biol. Chem.*, **54**, 567, 1990.
23. **Hirose, Y., Yamaoka, H., and Nakayama, M.,** Oxidation product of (-)-epicatechin under radical reaction, *J. Jpn. Oil Chem. Soc.*, **39**, 967, 1990.
24. **Hirose, Y., Yamaoka, H., and Nakayama, M.,** A novel quasi-dimeric oxidation product of (+)-catechin from lipid peroxidation, *J. Am. Oil Chem. Soc.*, **68**, 131, 1991.
25. **Nakayama, M. and Hirose, Y.,** Antioxidant activity of catechins and an approach to the antioxidant mechanism based on the oxidation products, *Foods Food Ingredients J. Jpn. (in Japanese)*, **161**, 1994.
26. **Sies, H.,** *Oxidative Stress*, Academic Press, London, 1987.
27. **Elias, P. S. and Cohen, A. J.,** *Radiation Chemistry of Major Food Components. Its Relevance to the Assessment of the Wholesomeness of*

Irradiated Foods, Elsevier/North Holland Press, Amsterdam, 1977.
28. **Terao, J., Piskula, M., and Yao, Q.**, Protective effect of epicatechin, epicatechin gallate, and quercetin on lipid peroxidation in phospholipid bilayers, *Arch. Biochem. Biophys.*, **308**, 278, 1994.
29. **Namiki, M. and Osawa, T.**, Antimutagenesis and anticarcinogenesis mechanism, in *Basic Life Science,* Plenum Press, New York, 1986, p. 131.
30. **Miura, S., Watanabe, J., Tomita, T., Sano, M., and Tomita, I.**, The inhibitory effects of tea polyphenols (flavan-3-ol derivatives) on Cu^{2+} mediated oxidative modification of low density lipoprotein, *Biol. Pharm. Bull.*, **17**, 1567, 1994.
31. **Miura, S., Watanabe, J., Sano, M., Tomita, T., Osawa, T., Hara, Y., and Tomita, I.**, Effects of various natural antioxidants on the Cu^{2+}-mediated oxidative modification of low density lipoprotein, *Biol. Pharm. Bull.*, **18**, 1, 1995.
32. **Sano, M., Takahashi, Y., Yoshino, K., Shimoi, K., Nakamura, Y., Tomita, I., Oguni, I., and Konomoto, H.**, Effect of tea (*Camellia sinensis* L.) on lipid peroxidation in rat liver and kidney: a comparison of green and black tea feeding, *Biol. Pharm. Bull.*, **18**, 1006, 1995.
33. **Kimura, Y., Okuda, H., Mori, K., Okuda, T., and Arichi, S.**, Effect of extracts of various kinds of tea on lipid metabolic injury in rats fed peroxidized oil, *Nippon Eiyo Shokuryo Gakkaishi (in Japanese)*, **37**, 223, 1984.
34. **Nanjo, F., Honda, M., Okushio, K., Matsumoto, N., Ishigaki, F., Ishigami, T., and Hara, Y.**, Effects of dietary tea catechins on alpha-tocopherol levels, lipid peroxidation, and erythrocyte deformability in rats fed on high palm oil and perilla oil diets, *Biol. Pharm. Bull.*, **16**, 1156, 1993.
35. **Yen, G. C. and Chen, H. Y.**, Antioxidant activity of various tea extracts in relation to their antimutagenicity, *J. Agr. Food Chem.*, **43**, 27, 1995.
36. **Halliwell, B. and Gutteridge, J. M. C.**, Role of free radicals and catalytic metal ions in human disease: an overview, *Meth. Enzymol.*, **186**, 1, 1990.
37. **Sai, K., Umemura, T., Takagi, A., Hasegawa, R., and Kurokawa, Y.**, The protective role of glutathione, cysteine and vitamin C against oxidative DNA damage induced in rat kidney by potassium bromate, *Jpn. J. Cancer Res.*, **83**, 45, 1992.
38. **Takagi, A., Sai, K., Uemura, T., Hasegawa, R., and Kurokawa, Y.**, Relationship between hepatic peroxisome proliferation and 8-hydroxydeoxyguanosine formation in liver DNA of rats following long-term exposure to three peroxisome proliferators; di (2-ethylhexyl) phthalate, aluminium clofibrate and simfibrate, *Cancer Lett.*, **53**, 33, 1990.
39. **Kasai, H. and Nishimura, S.**, Hydroxylation of deoxyguanosine at the C8 position by ascorbic acid and other reducing agents, *Nucleic Acids Res.*, **12**, 2137, 1984.
40. **Floyd, R. A.**, The role of 8-oxodeoxyguanosine levels in carcinogenesis, *Carcinogenesis*, **11**, 1447, 1990.
41. **Chung, F.-L. and Xu, L.**, Increased 8-oxodeoxy-guanosine levels in lung DNA of A/J mice and F344 rats treated with the tobacco-specific nitrosamine 4-(methylnitrosamine)-1-(3-pyridyl)-1-butanone, *Carcinogenesis*, **13**, 1269, 1992.

42. **Xu, Y., Ho, C. T., Amin, S. G., Han, C., and Chung, F. L.,** Inhibition of tobacco-specific nitrosamine-induced lung tumorigenesis in A/J mice by green tea and its major polyphenol as antioxidants, *Cancer Res.*, **52**, 3875, 1992.
43. **Umemura, T., Sai, K., Takagi, A., Hasegawa, R., and Kurokawa, Y.,** Formation of 8-hydroxydeoxyguanosine (8-OH-dG) in rat kidney DNA after intraperitoneal administration of ferric nitrilotriacetate (Fe-NTA), *Carcinogenesis*, **11**, 345, 1990.
44. **Wei, H. C. and Frenkel, K.,** Relationship of oxidative events and DNA oxidation in SENCAR mice to *in vivo* promoting activity of phorbol ester-type tumor promoters, *Carcinogenesis*, **14**, 1195, 1993.
45. **Hasegawa, R., Chujo, T., Sai-kato, K., Uemura, T., Tanimura, A., and Kurokawa, Y.,** Preventive effects of green tea against liver oxidative DNA damage and hepatotoxicity in rats treated with 2-Nitropropane, *Food Chem. Toxicol.*, **33**, 961, 1995.
46. **Inagake, M., Yamane, T., Kitao, Y., Oya, K., Matsumoto, H., Kikuoka, N., Nakatani, H., Takahashi, T., Nishimura, H., and Iwashima, A.,** Inhibition of 1,2-dimethylhydrazine-induced oxidative DNA damage by green tea extract in rat, *Jpn. J. Cancer Res.*, **86**, 1106, 1995.

Chapter 5

METABOLISM OF TEA POLYPHENOLS

H. Takahashi and M. Ninomiya

TABLE OF CONTENTS

I. Introduction
II. Administration of Tea Polyphenols
III. Absorption of Tea Polyphenols from Intestine
IV. Effects of Tea Polyphenols on the Digestive Tract
V. Organ Distribution of Tea Polyphenols
VI. Excretion of Tea Polyphenols
VII. Metabolism of Tea Polyphenols
    A. Metabolites in Urine
    B. Metabolites in Feces
    C. Metabolites in Bile
    D. Metabolic Pathway
VIII. Toxicity of Polyphenols
References

I. INTRODUCTION

Recently, many researches have been focused on the preventive effect of adult disease using green tea polyphenols, decaffeinated green tea polyphenols, and purified compounds. However, for food chemical and pharmaceutical application of tea polyphenols, e.g., for cancer prevention, therapy of hypocholesterolemia, or prevention of hypertension, it is necessary to know the metabolic fate of tea polyphenols in humans as well as in experimental animals. Also, in order to decide the dose, the concentration of tea polyphenols in blood and tissue through which they act must be made clear. The metabolism of tea polyphenols, however, has not been elucidated completely. The reason for this is shortage of experimental data due to the difficulty of the synthesis of the polyphenols labeled with an isotope. Recently, however, the analysis of polyphenols has been eased by means of the HPLC or GLC method. Several metabolic products from tea polyphenols in blood, urine, and feces have thus been isolated and their structures, determined to be useful for making the metabolism of tea polyphenols clear.

II. ADMINISTRATION OF TEA POLYPHENOLS

A cup of green tea infusion generally contains about 50-100 mg of tea polyphenols. In the experiments, a dried preparation of green tea extracts was administrated to experimental animals and young male volunteers at a dose of 0.5 or 1.2 g per day (Table 1 and 2). These doses correspond to 0.3-0.7 g polyphenols per day. In the case of using green tea leaf powder for hyperlipidemia, the dose was also adjusted to stand for 0.6 g tea polyphenols per day [4]. Several researchers reported that daily intake of 0.5 g tea polyphenols resulted in an increase of HDL-cholesterol and a decrease in blood pressure [1]. No defective symptom was observed even when the dose of 0.7 g polyphenols per day was continued for a month for healthy men carried out as a control test [2]. The daily dose above is a useful reference in determining therapeutic dose of tea polyphenols for hyperlipidemia, cardiovascular disease, renal failure, etc.

Table 1
Administration of Green Tea Polyphenols to Human Volunteers

Sample	Amount of supplement (g/day)	Duration (days)	Subjects	Reference
Green tea polyphenols*	1.2	28	Healthy volunteers	Okubo et al. [1]
	0.5	84	Healthy volunteers	Kanaya et al. [2]
	0.4	84	Renal failure patients	Yokozawa et al. [3]

*SUNPHENON^R (Taiyo Kagaku Co., Ltd.)

Table 2
Administration of Green Tea Polyphenols to Experimental Animals

Sample	Dose	Period (days)	Animals	Items	Reference
Green tea polyphenols	0.5 g/kg	28	rats	hypercholesterolemia	Matsuda [4]
	0.5 g/l (drinking water)	50	mice	skin tumor	Wang [5]
	0.2 or 2 g/kg	24 hr	rats	chromosome aberration	Ito [6]
	0.01 or 0.1% (drinking water)	112	rats	colon cancer	Yamane [7]
Green tea polyphenols*	0.1, 0.25, or 0.5 (mg/rat/day)	14	rats	renal failure	Yokozawa [8]
Green tea polyphenols	1.2 or 3.6 mg (twice weekly)	21 weeks	mice	skin tumor	Huang [9]
	0.05, 0.1, or 0.2%	5 times	rats	hepatic injury	Hayashi [10]
	0.2% (wt/vol)	30	mice	antioxidant	Khan [11]
	0.2% (wt/vol)	30	mice	skin radiation	Agarwal [12]
	5 mg/mouse	once	mice	neoplasia	Katiyar [13]
	0.63 or 1.25%	30	mice	skin cancer	Wang [14]

*SUNPHENON^R (Taiyo Kagaku Co., Ltd.)

Matsuda and his colleagues [4] gave green tea polyphenols to hypercholesterolemic rats at a dose of 0.5 g per kg body weight. For prevention of azoxymethane (AOM)-induced colon cancer, the drinking water containing 0.01 or 0.1% green tea extracts (SUNPHENON[R], Taiyo Kagaku Co., Ltd., polyphenol content, 60%) was given to rats for 16 weeks [7]. But, no papers have been reported so far on the occurrence of any toxic symptom by administration of tea polyphenols.

III. ABSORPTION OF TEA POLYPHENOLS FROM INTESTINE

There has been only a little information about the absorption of tea polyphenols from intestine and its level in blood. In 60 min after oral administration of 200 mg per kg body weight in rats, 30-40% of (+)-catechin ([U-^{14}C] catechin), one of green tea's polyphenols, was found to be absorbed from the small intestine [15]. The maximum level of radioactivity in blood was observed in 1-2 hr after the administration. These data show that (+)-catechin is readily absorbed from small intestine suggesting that other tea polyphenols would be similarly absorbed from small intestine.

IV. EFFECTS OF TEA POLYPHENOLS ON THE DIGESTIVE TRACT

Polyphenols and related compounds have been reported to reduce the digestibility of certain nutrients which results in growth depression [16]. Recently, it was reported that amylase activity was suppressed by oral administration of several tannins including tea polyphenols, and the plasma glucose level of chickens was found to be suppressed [17]. Cholecystokinin (CCK) is an important substance to stimulate both pancreatic enzymes secretion and gall bladder contraction. We investigated the levels of plasma CCK and pancreatic enzyme activities after administration of tea polyphenols to rats [18]. The plasma CCK level was significantly increased (Figure 1). Trypsin activity was also increased. However, intestinal amylase activity was depressed by tea polyphenols (Figure 2).

Certain components of polyphenols have been reported to inhibit absorption of iron in diet. Dislar and his colleagues [19] suggested that tannin in tea infusion gives rise to reduction in iron absorption in malignant anemic women.

V. ORGAN DISTRIBUTION OF TEA POLYPHENOLS

Kurita and his research group investigated the distribution of (+)-[U-^{14}C] catechin administered to rats at a dose of 200 mg per kg [15]. In 1 hr after the administration, a high radioactivity was found in kidney, liver, skin, lung, and heart blood. But, it was not detected in brain, adrenal glands, heart, muscle, testis, and ovary. Even 24 hr later, a high radioactivity was still observed in liver, lung, adrenal glands, spleen, testis, salivary gland, and bone marrow. But, no radioactivity was detected in any tissue 48 hr later, suggesting that tea polyphenols have no particular organotropism.

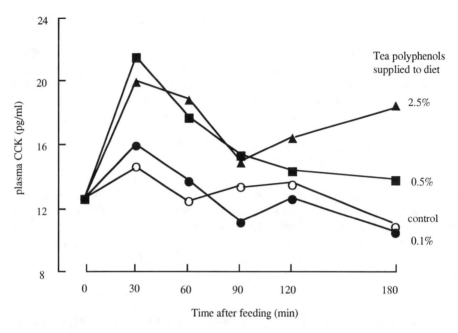

Figure 1. Time course of the effect of tea polyphenols on concentration of cholecystokinin (CCK) in plasma of rats. Rats were given a single diet of 3.8 g with or without polyphenols via an orogastric tube. Each point represents the mean of five observations. Reproduced from Yang et al. (1992) [18] by permission of Japan Society for Bioscience, Biotechnology, and Agrochemistry, Tokyo.

VI. EXCRETION OF TEA POLYPHENOLS

Matsumoto and his colleagues have reported that when (-)-epigallocatechin gallate (EGCg) was administered to rats at a dose of 50 mg per head, 40% of the EGCg was excreted to feces in the intact state while in urine and bile, no EGCg was detected [20]. However, in our experiments, 1.8-4% of EGCg was detected in urine of the rats which were administered with 100 mg EGCg per head. This discrepancy seems to be attributed to the difference in the amount of dosage.

It was also reported that rats were administered (+)-catechin at a dose of 200 mg per kg body weight, the excretion of radioactivity of [U-^{14}C] into urine and feces was 31-32% and 50-60%, respectively [21]. The respiratory excretion was, therefore, estimated to be 7-9% of the total activity. Also, the cumulative biliary excretion of the radioactivity of (+)-[U-14C] catechin was estimated to be 31-32% of the total activity in the case of male rats when orally administered. Also, 85% of biliary excretion of (+)-catechin was presumed to be that reabsorbed from intestine [15].

VII. METABOLISM OF TEA POLYPHENOLS

A. METABOLITES IN URINE

Garo [22] reported that orally administered (-)-epicatechin and related compounds in humans were excreted 20% of the orally administered

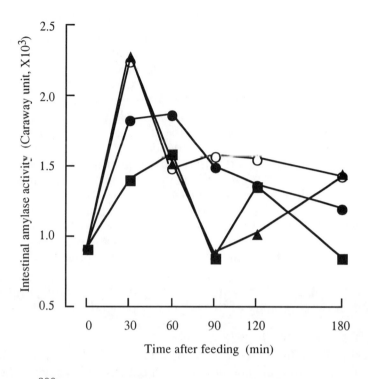
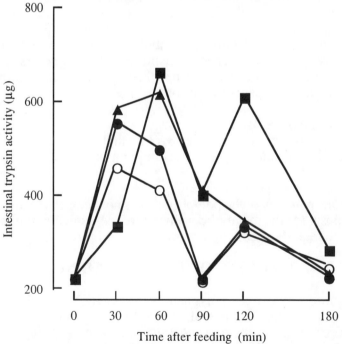

Figure 2. Time course of activities of intestinal amylase and trypsin of rats after supplement of diet with or without tea polyphenol. The diet was given as a single meal at 3.8 g via an orogastric tube. Each point represents the mean of five observations.
O, control; ●, 0.1%; ■, 0.5%; ▲, 2.5%. Reproduced from Yang et al. (1992) [18] by permission of Japan Society for Bioscience, Biotechnology, and Agrochemistry, Tokyo.

(-)-epicatechin. The structure of the excreted compound was not changed. Whereas in guinea pigs given intraperitoneally, the structure of excreted (+)-catechin was unchanged at 65%. Griffiths [23] reported that a dose of 50 mg of (+)-catechin per head to rats by oral administration gave rise to such metabolites as m-hydroxyphenylpropionic acid and m-hydroxyhippuric acid in the urine. The results suggested that the formation of these metabolites was the result by the action of gut microflora, because a high oral dose of antibiotics suppressed their formation. The fact that the amount of (-)-epicatechin in feces was much smaller than that in urine is evidence that (-)-epicatechin and related compounds are readily absorbed through the intestinal wall. Also, Das and Griffiths [21] found that m-hydroxyphenylpropionic acids, δ-(3-hydroxyphenyl)-γ-valerolactone and δ-(3,4-dihydroxyphenyl)-γ-valerolactone appeared as additional metabolites. Hachett and his colleagues [24] showed that when [^{14}C]-(+)-catechin was administered to rats, these three compounds in urine accounted for 84% of the total ^{14}C that was estimated by the radio scanning method for TLC separates of the metabolites. The conjugated compounds were a glucuronide of (+)-catechin and a glucuronide and a sulfate of 3'-O-methyl-(+)-catechin which were identified by applying specific enzymes and chromatography of the aglycons liberated.

B. METABOLITES IN FECES

(+)-Catechin is metabolized by various bacteria in large intestine to m-hydroxyphenylpropionic acid and m-hydroxyhippuric acid. They are, however, readily absorbed from gut tube. The reason for this observation was that m-hydroxyphenylpropionic acids found in feces was very small in amount [23]. It is now known that (+)-catechin is metabolized mainly to hydroxyphenyl-valeric acids by intestinal microorganisms in the *in vitro* test [25]. Two diarylpropan-2-ol metabolites have been isolated from the incubation mixture of (+)-catechin with rat's cecal microflora [26].

C. METABOLITES IN BILE

Shaw and Griffiths have reported that 3'-O-methyl-(+)- catechin glucuronide is a major metabolic product of (+)-catechin in rat bile [27].

D. METABOLIC PATHWAY

The metabolic pathway of tea polyphenols has not been clarified completely yet, but a proposal for the metabolic pathways of (+)-catechin in rats has been reported by Miura and his colleagues as shown in Figure 3 [28].

VIII. TOXICITY OF TEA POLYPHENOLS

The lethal dose of green tea polyphenols (SUNPHENON^R, Taiyo Kagaku Co., Ltd., 60% polyphenols) was estimated to be 3.09 g per kg for female and more than 5.0 g per kg for male of *ddy* mice. In our oral dosing study using rats with the daily dose of 15 and 75 mg per kg for 88 days, no toxic symptoms were observed for the administration of green tea polyphenols.

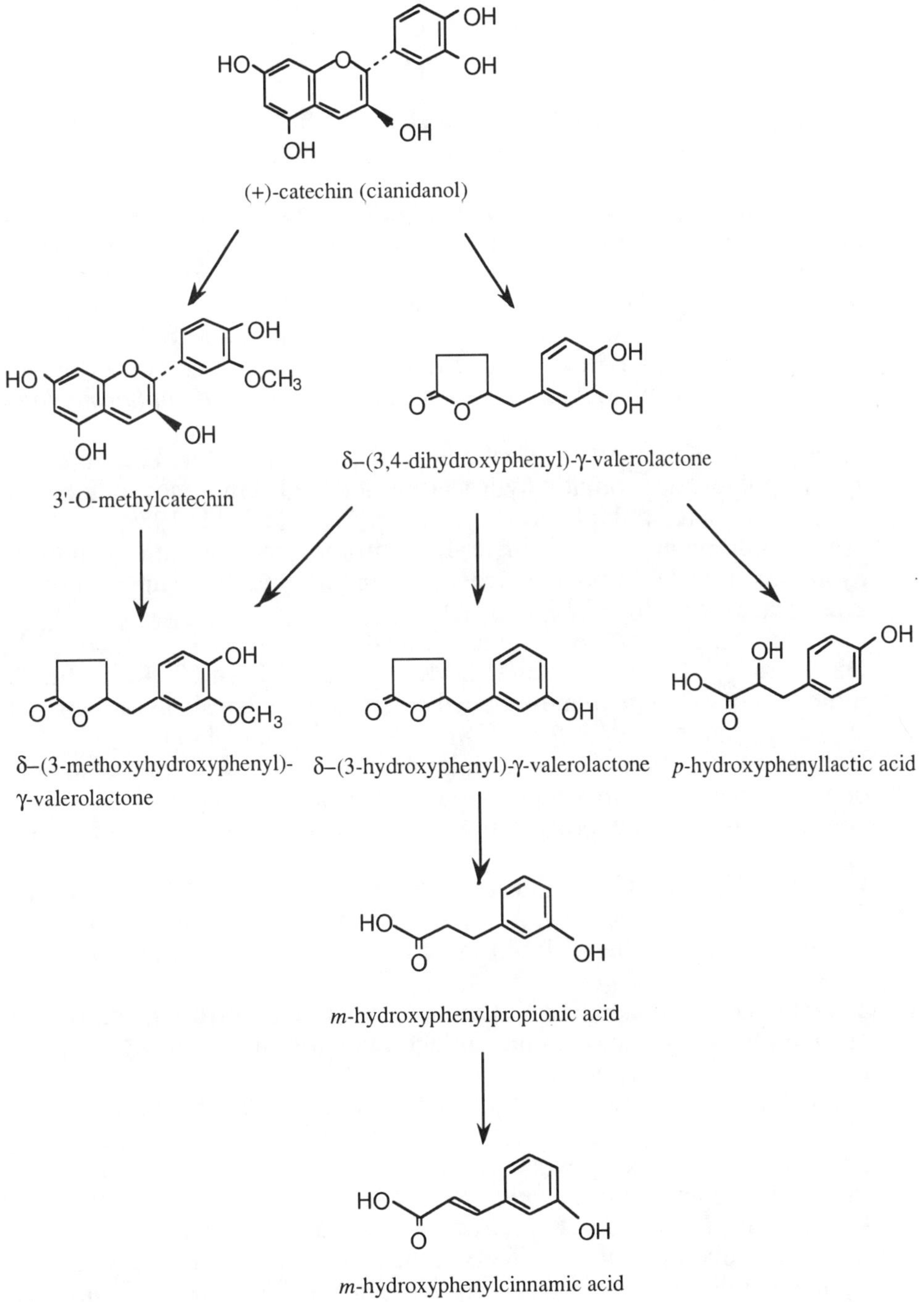

Figure 3. Proposed metabolic pathways of (+)-catechin.
Reproduced from Miura et al. (1983) [28] by permission of The Japanese Society of Pharmacometrics, Sendai.

REFERENCES

1. Okubo, T., Ishihara, N., Oura, A., Serit, M., Kim, M., Yamamoto, T., and Mitsuoka, T., *In vivo* effects of tea polyphenol intake on human intestinal microflora and metabolism, *Biosci. Biotech. Biochem.*, **56**, 588, 1992.
2. Kanaya, S., Goto, K., Hara, Y., and Hospital, S. M. G., The physiological effects of tea catechins on human volunteers, in *International Tea Symposium*, 1993, p 314.
3. Yokozawa, T., Shibata, T., Oura, H., Hasegawa, M., Sakanaka, S., Ishigaki, S., and Kim, M., Effect of green tea polyphenols on the hemodialysis patients suffering from uremic toxin formation, *Nippon Nogeikagaku Kaishi (in Japanaese)*, **68**, 157, 1994.
4. Matsuda, H., Chisaka, T., Kubomura, Y., Yamahara, J., Sawada, T., Fujimura, H., and Kimura, H., Effects of crude drugs on experimental hypercholesterolemia. I.Tea and its active principles, *J. Ethnopharmcology*, **17**, 213, 1986.
5. Wang, Z. Y., Khan, W. A., Bickers, D. R., and Mukhtar, H., Protection against polycyclic aromatic hydrocarbon-induced skin tumor initiation in mice by green tea polyphenols, *Carcinogenesis*, **10**, 411, 1989.
6. Ito, Y., Ohonishi, S., and Fujie, K., Chromosome aberrations induced by aflatoxin B1 in rat bone marrow cells *in vivo* and their suppression by green tea, *Mutat. Res.*, **222**, 253, 1989.
7. Yamane, T., Hagiwara, N. and Tateishi, M., Akachi, S., Kim, M., Okuzumi, J., Kitao, Y., Inagaki, M., Kuwata, K., and Takahashi, T., Inhibition of azoxymethane-induced colon carcinogenesis in rat by green tea polyphenol fraction, *Jpn J. Cancer Res.*, **82**, 1336, 1991.
8. Yokozawa, T., Oura, H., Sakanaka, S., and Kim, M., Effect of tannins in green tea on the urinary methylguanidine excretion in rats indicating a possible radical scavenging action, *Biosci. Biotech. Biochem.*, **56**, 896, 1992.
9. Huang, M-T., Ho, C-T., Yaung, Z-Y., Ferraro, T-F., Innegan-Olive, T., Lou, Y-R., and Conney, A. H., Inhibitory effect of topical application of a green tea polyphenol fraction on tumor initiation and promotion in mice skin, *Carcinogenesis*, **13**, 947, 1992.
10. Hayashi, M., Yamazoe, H., Yamaguchi, Y., and Kunitomo, M., Effects of green tea on galactosamine-induced hepatic injury in rats, *Nippon Yakugaku Zasshi (in Japanese)*, **100**, 391, 1992.
11. Khan, S. G., Katiyar, S. K., Agarwal, R., and Mukhtar, H., Enhancement of antioxidant and phase II enzymes by oral feeding of green tea polyphenols in drinking water to SKH-1 hairless mice: possible role in cancer chemoprevention, *Cancer Res.*, **52**, 4050, 1992.
12. Agarwal, R., Katiyar, S. K., Khan, S. G., and Mukhtar, H., Protection against B radiation-induced effects in the skin of SKH-1 hairless mice by a polyphenolic fraction isolated from green tea, *Photochem. Photobiol.*, **58**, 695, 1993.
13. Katiyar, S. K., Agarwal, R., and Mukhtar, H., Protective effects of green tea polyphenols administered by oral intubation against chemical carcinogen-induced forestomach and pulmonary neoplasia in A/J mice, *Cancer Lett.*, **73**, 167, 1993.

14. **Wang, Z. Y., Huang, M-T., Lou, Y-R., Xie, J-G., Reuhl, K. R., Newmark, H. L., Ho, C-T., Yang, C. S., and Conney, A. H.,** Inhibitory effects of black tea, green tea, decaffeinated black tea, and decaffeinated green tea on ultraviolet B light-induced skin carcinogenesis in 7,12-dimethylbenz[a]anthracene-initiated SKH-1 mice, *Cancer Res.*, **54**, 3428, 1994.
15. **Kurita, N., Miura, S., Hamada, T., Satomi, O., and Midorikawa, T.,** Metabolic fate of cianidanol (1) absorption, distribution and excretion in rats, *Oyo Yakuri (in Japanese)*, **25**, 993, 1983.
16. **Mahmood, S. and Smitharrd, R.,** A comparison of effects of body weight and feed intake on digestion in broiler cockerels with effects of tannins, *Bri. J. Nutr.*, **70**, 701, 1993.
17. **Matsumoto, N., Ishigami, F., Ishigaki, A., Iwashina, H., and Hara, Y.,** Reduction of blood glucose levels by tea catechin, *Biosci. Biotech. Biochem.*, **57**, 525, 1993.
18. **Yang, S. I., Takahashi, H., Kobayashi, T., Fujiki, M., Kim, M., and Yamamoto, T.,** Effect of tea polyphenols on the digestion activity, *Nippon Nogeikagaku Kaishi (in Japanese)*, **66**, 62, 1992.
19. **Dislar, P. B., Lynch, S. R., Charlton, R. W., Torrance, J. D., Bothwell, T. H., Walker, R. B., and Mayet, F.,** The effect of tea on iron absorption, *Gut*, **16**, 193, 1975.
20. **Matsumoto, N., Tono-oka, F., Ishigaki, A., Okushino, K., and Hara, Y.,** The fate of (-)-epicgallocatechin gallate (EGCg) in the digestive tract of rats, in *Proceedings of the International Symposium on Tea Science,* Kurofune Printing Co. Ltd., Shizuoka, 1991, p 253.
21. **Das, N. P. and Griffiths, L. A.,** Studies on flavonoid metabolism, *Biochem. J.*, **115**, 831, 1969.
22. **Gero, E.,** Etude de l'elimination urinaire de l'epicatechine, *Arch. Int. Phisiol (in French)*, **54**, 201, 1946.
23. **Griffiths, L. A.,** Studies on flavonoid metabolism, *Biochem. J.*, **92**, 173, 1964.
24. **Hachett, A. M., Shaw, I. C., and Griffiths, L. A.,** 3'-O-methyl-(+)catechin glucronide and 3'-O-methyl-(+)catechin sulphate: new urinary metabolites of (+)catechin in the rats and marmoset, *Experientia*, **38**, 538, 1982.
25. **Scheline, R. R.,** The metabolism of (+)-catechin to hydroxyphenyvaleric acids by the intestinal microflora, *Biochem. Biophys. Acta*, **222**, 228, 1970.
26. **Groenewoud, G. and Hundt, H. K. L.,** The microbial metabilism of (+)-catechin to two novel diarylpropan-2-ol metabolites *in vitro*, *Xenobiotica*, **14**, 711, 1984.
27. **Shaw, I. C. and Griffiths, L. A.,** Identification of the major biliary metabolite of (+)-catechin in the rat, *Xenobiotica*, **10**, 905, 1980.
28. **Miura, S., Hamada, T., Satomi, O., Midorikawa, T., and Kurita, N.,** Metabolic fate of cianidanol (3) *in vivo* and *in vitro* metabolism in rats, *Oyo Yakuri (in Japanese)*, **25**, 1015, 1983.

Chapter 6

CANCER CHEMOPREVENTION BY GREEN TEA POLYPHENOLS

M. Kim and M. Masuda

TABLE OF CONTENTS

I. Introduction
II. Epidemiological Studies on the Relationship Between Tea and Cancer
III. Laboratory Studies on the Relation Between Green Tea and Cancer
IV. Chemopreventive Effect of Green Tea Polyphenols on Carcinogenesis in Rats
    A. Materials and Methods
        1. Animals and Diets
        2. Chemicals
        3. Experimental Protocol
        4. Histological Examination
        5. Statistical Analysis
    B. Results
        1. Body Weights
        2. Colon Tumors
        3. Inhibition by GTP
V. Conclusions
References

I. INTRODUCTION

It is a general concept that carcinogenesis proceeds stepwise through the three stages of the so-called initiation, promotion, and progression stages. The initiation stage is essentially irreversible in which genetic changes occur in the gene(s) to control differentiation. The promotion stage leads to the development of visible nonmalignant lesions. Some of these premalignant lesions develop into malignant neoplasms, and this process is the progression stage [1]. Carcinogenesis, a multistep process, requires both initiating and promoting substances for induction or its development of cancer. Regarding the above-mentioned processes, a number of studies have demonstrated the preventive effect of naturally occurring compounds against tumor induction and its growth. The effective compounds are referred to as cancer chemopreventive agents. Chemoprevention of cancer may make it possible to control the initiation and promotion events occurring during the process of neoplastic development by administration of such effective natural compounds.

    Chemoprevention differs from cancer treatment in that the goal of prevention is to lower the rate of cancer incidence. For these strategies, the chemicals with anticarcinogenic effect should be non-toxic and if possible, they should be those originated from our foods such as fruits, vegetables, and beverages. Foods are complex materials which are taken daily in large quantities. If one makes an extreme argument, foods are the material to provide medical and health benefits together with their nutritive compounds. During the past few decades, much attention has thus been paid to define the relationship between particular food ingredients and health benefits. The results obtained by the efforts, especially that of epidemiological investigations, have shown that some food ingredients play an important role in reducing the risk of development of a number of human cancers.

Many reports regarding cancer chemoprevention have been published, and the National Cancer Institute of the U.S.A. has adopted a systematic approach to support the development of new chemopreventive agents [2]. In Japan, epidemiological studies on the relationship between green tea and cancer have shown that the people who have taken green tea infusion more frequently were significantly lower in the risk for stomach cancer. This statistical result was particularly true in Shizuoka Prefecture, a famous district for production of green tea in Japan [3]. These results suggest a big possibility for green tea as the most potential natural cancer chemopreventive agent.

II. EPIDEMIOLOGICAL STUDIES ON THE RELATIONSHIP BETWEEN TEA AND CANCER

A search for the preventive effect of certain chemical compounds on the target disease can be reliably accomplished by epidemiological studies. In 1989, the International Agency for Research on Cancer Working Group reviewed the results of epidemiological studies in the relation of tea consumption with the occurrence of human cancers [4]. The review was carried out based on the literature available. However, the review did not show any general conclusion regarding the relationship between tea consumption and cancer risk because of inadequate analysis and inconsistent results.

In 1993, Yang and his research group reviewed and discussed the results obtained in more recent studies [5]. As can be seen from Table 1, a general overview on the relationship between tea and human cancer made it difficult to deduce an emphasized conclusion.

However, the complexity with a similar tendency still exists. For example, some research groups reported a preventive effect of tea on lung cancer, while others reported negative effects regarding cancer of the same organ. The contradictory results of these studies may be ascribed to: 1) differences in the lifestyle of the subjects including the problems about whether they were smoker and drinker or not, 2) diversity of cancer in different site organs, and 3) difference in the type of tea tested, such as green tea, black tea, and oolong tea. In general, black tea is the predominant tea consumed in western countries, while green tea is the major tea consumed in Japan. In China, green tea and oolong tea both are consumed. Also, oolong tea is consumed in the southern part of China and recently in Japan. 4) In addition, the differences in tea drinking habits at normal temperatures (35-47°C) and hot temperatures (55-67°C) are known as important factors for occurrence of human cancer rather than the effect of chemicals of the tea. For example, the study in Kazakhstan where tea is consumed as a hot drink, suggested that green tea was a cancer risk factor [6]. As a consequence, these variations would further complicate the study of the effect of tea consumption and cancer. Therefore, a precise epidemiological study in relation to tea consumption and cancer chemoprevention by using

Table 1
Epidemiology Studies: Relationship Between Tea Drinking and Human Cancer [5]

Organ	Association of tea drinking to cancer	Number and type of studies
Bladder and urinary tract	No relationship	1 ecological study
		2 cohort studies
		16 case-control studies
Breast	Positive	1 ecological study
	No relationship	5 case-control studies
	Negative	1 ecological study
Colon and rectum	Positive	1 ecological study
		1 cohort study
		1 case-control study
	No relationship	1 cohort study
		5 case-control studies
	Negative	3 case-control studies
Esophagus	Positive	3 ecological studies
		5 case-control studies (with high-temperature tea)
	No relationship	1 ecological study
		4 case-control studies (with normal-temperature tea)
		2 case-control studies
Kidney	Positive	1 cohort study
		1 case-control study
	No relationship	1 ecological study
		5 case-control studies
Liver	No relationship	1 ecological study
		1 cohort study
		1 case-control study
	Negative	1 ecological study
Lung	Positive	1 ecological study
		1 cohort study
		1 case-control study
	Negative	1 ecological study
Nasopharynx	No relationship	3 case-control studies
Pancreas	Positive	1 case-control study
	No relationship	3 cohort studies
		7 case-control studies
	Negative	1 cohort study
		1 case-control study
Stomach	Positive	1 cohort study
		1 case-control study
	No relationship	7 case-control studies
	Negative	2 ecological studies
		2 case-control studies
Uterus	Negative	2 ecological studies

human clinical trials will be indispensable. Concerning this problem, the results of the epidemiological studies carried out on green tea infusion as drinks under the normal condition, showed some noteworthy facts.

A case control study in Kyushu, Japan, showed that individuals who had consumed green tea in larger quantities were lower in the risk for gastric cancer [7]. The study in the Shizuoka Prefecture area, performed focusing on stomach cancer, revealed a lower incidence than the national average. In Korea, the chemopreventive effect of green tea among cigarette smokers was examined using sister chromatid exchange (SCE) frequencies in peripheral lymphocytes as a mutagenic marker. The frequencies of SCE rate were significantly elevated in smokers, but SCE rate in smokers who consumed green tea infusion daily (2-3 cups/day) was reduced, implying that green tea can block a cigarette-induced increase in SCE frequency [8].

These observations in recent studies make it clear that drinking green tea is distinctly beneficial in reducing cancer risk.

III. LABORATORY STUDIES ON THE RELATION BETWEEN GREEN TEA AND CANCER

Since epidemiological study involves various factors which may bring inexplicable results, experiments using animal models will be necessary to employ the conditions that make the chemopreventive effect clear. This is of course true for examination of the effect of green tea. A number of researchers have studied the effects of green tea infusion, tea polyphenol fractions, or their purified components, especially (-)-epigallocatechin gallate (EGCg,) for the esophagus, forestomach, duodenum, small intestine, colon, skin, lung, liver, pancreas, and mammary gland using several rodent models such as mouse, rat, and hamster. The inhibitory effect of green tea against tumorigenesis was evidenced in the following experiments.

Esophagus - The oral administration of 2% tea infusion as the sole source of drinking water inhibited esophageal tumorigenesis which was induced by N-nitrosomethylbenzylamine (NMBzA) in rats. The tumor incidence was depressed by 26-53%, and the tumor multiplicity was reduced by 58-75% [9]. The oral feeding of tea infusion also inhibited esophageal tumor formation which was induced by precursors of NMBzA or by N-nitrososarcosine in mice.

Forestomach - The oral administration of 1.2% green tea infusion to mice significantly inhibited benzo(a)pyrene (BP) or N-nitrosodiethylamine (NDEA)-induced forestomach tumorigenesis [10]. The oral feeding of green tea infusion also inhibited forestomach tumor formation induced by precursors of NMBzA or N-nitrososarcosine in mice.

Glandular stomach - The solution of 0.05% EGCg given per os (p. o.) inhibited N-methyl-N'-nitro-N-nitrosoguanidine (MNNG)-induced carcinogenesis of the glandular stomach in rats. The percentage of tumor bearing rats in the group treated with MNNG plus EGCg was 31% while that of the control group was 62% [11].

Duodenum - The oral feeding of 0.005% EGCg in drinking water to mice with MNNG inhibited tumor formation in duodenum [12].

Skin - The topical application of green tea polyphenols or EGCg to mouse skin has shown to result in protection from tumor initiation by 7, 12-dimethyl benzanthracene (DMBA) and benzopyrenediolepoxide (BPDE) [13, 14]. The topical application of green tea polyphenols also inhibited ultraviolet radiation-induced skin tumorigenesis. It is a really surprising fact that even the oral feeding of green tea polyphenols inhibited skin tumor initiation induced by DMBA, skin tumor promotion by 12-O-tetradecanoylphorbol-1, 3-acetate (TPA), and tumorigenesis by ultraviolet rays [15, 16].

Lung - The oral administration of green tea infusion (0.65 or 1.25%) as the sole source of drinking water to mice inhibited NDEA-induced lung tumorigenesis [17]. Similar results were observed that 2% green tea solution or EGCg in drinking water inhibited 45 or 35%, respectively, of the lung tumor multiplicity induced by a tobacco carcinogen, 4-methylnitrosoamino-3-pyridyl-1-butanone (NNK) [18]. It was also reported that the oral feeding of 0.05% green tea polyphenols to ddY mice resulted in a 60% reduction of 4-nitroquinoline-1-oxide-induced lung tumorigenesis [19].

Liver - The administration of 2.5% green tea leaves to the diet of rats produced a significant inhibition of NDEA-induced hepatocarcinogenesis [20]. It was also observed that a solution of either 0.05% or 0.1% EGCg was effective to inhibit spontaneous hepatoma development in C3H/HeN mice.

Pancreas - In a carcinogenesis model induced with N-nitroso-bis (2-oxopropyl) amine (BOP) to Syrian golden hamsters, green tea polyphenols (500 mg/kg per day) resulted in reduction of the incidence of pancreatic carcinogenesis [21].

Mammary gland - A polyphenol-aluminum complex (0.2%) added to the diet inhibited the spontaneous mammary tumor incidence in the experiment using C3H/HeN mice which were easy to give rise to spontaneous mammary tumor formation [22].

IV. CHEMOPREVENTIVE EFFECT OF GREEN TEA POLYPHENOLS ON COLON CARCINOGENESIS IN RATS

Green tea polyphenols have clearly shown antitumor activities in various organs of several animal models, as described above. The effect of green tea polyphenols on colon cancer was also evidenced. This fact is very important because of a rapid increase in the incidence of large intestinal cancer recently in Japan.

As mentioned above, EGCg inhibited the promotion stage of duodenal carcinogenesis which was induced by N-methyl-N'-nitro-N-nitrosoguanidine [12]. This fact suggested the possibility that green tea polyphenols might be effective to prevent carcinogenesis of the alimentary tract. In addition, green tea polyphenols have been shown to inhibit the growth of intestinal clostridia *in vitro* and *in vivo* [23, 24]. The bacteria have been considered to be associated with the biotransformation of various ingested or endogenously formed compounds to be carcinogenic such as N-nitroso compounds or aromatic steroids. These observations led us to study the influence of green tea polyphenols on colon carcinogenesis (Figure 1). The inhibitory effect of green tea polyphenols on colon carcinogenesis induced by azoxymethane (AOM) in rats is thus described in detail below [25].

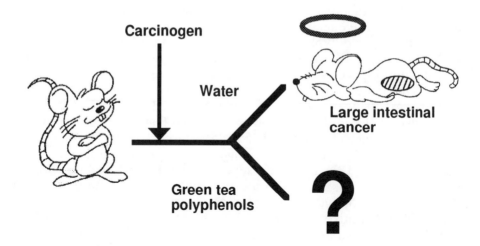

Figure 1. Experimental design to evidence the inhibitory effect of green tea polyphenols on large intestine cancer.

A. MATERIALS AND METHODS
1. Animals and Diets
Eight-week-old Fisher rats were purchased from Japan SLC Inc. (Shizuoka, Japan) and given free access to drinking water and standard laboratory chow MF (Oriental Yeast Co., Tokyo, Japan).

2. Chemicals
AOM was purchased from Sigma Chemical Co. (St. Louis, MO, U.S.A.), and kept at -80°C before use. Green tea polyphenols (GTP) used in this study was SUNPHENON[R], a product of Taiyo Kagaku Co., Ltd. (Yokkaichi, Japan). It contains 75% of polyphenolic compounds, which consisted of six catechin derivatives: (+)-catechin, (-)-epicatechin, (-)-epicatechin gallate, (-)-gallocatechin, (-)-epigallocatechin, and (-)-epigallocatechin gallate.

3. Experimental Protocol
AOM was dissolved in 0.9% NaCl solution and injected s.c. at a dosage of 7.4 mg/kg body weight once a week for the first 10 weeks. In a week after the last AOM treatment, the treated rats were divided into three groups: AOM-control (26 rats), AOM-GTP1 (26 rats), and AOM-GTP2 (25 rats). The AOM-control group received tap water throughout the experiment. The AOM-GTP1 and AOM-GTP2 groups received 0.01 and 0.1% GTP, respectively, dissolved in tap water as drinking water from week 11 to 26. On the other hand, 3 groups of 10 rats each without AOM treatment — i.e., a control group (tap water throughout the experiment) and GTP1 and GTP2 (0.01% and 0.1% GTP, respectively, in tap water) — were prepared as the counterparts of the above AOM-treated groups. Rats in these referrence groups were also injected s.c. for the first 10 weeks, but with 0.9% NaCl solution containing no AOM.

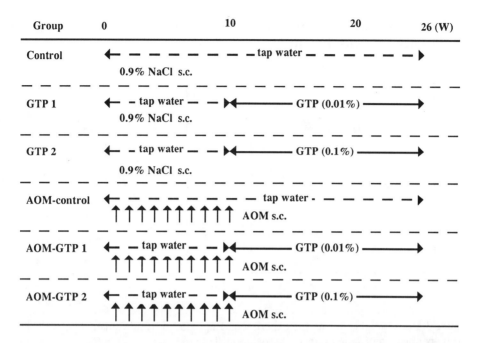

Figure 2. Experimental schedule for the inhibitory test of green tea polyphenols fraction (GTP) against AOM-induced colon carcinogenesis. AOM was injected s.c. at a dosage of 7.4 mg/kg body weight once a week for the first 10 weeks. Rats received GTP in the drinking water from week 11. The experiment was terminated at week 26. AOM-control, AOM-treated rats without GTP; AOM-GTP1, AOM-treated rats with 0.01% GTP; AOM-GTP2, AOM-treated rats with 0.1% GTP; Control, untreated rats (i.e., no AOM treatment) without GTP; GTP1, untreated rats with 0.01% GTP; GTP2, untreated rats with 0.1% GTP. Reproduced from Yamane et al. (1991) [25] by permission of Japan Cancer Association, Tokyo.

4. Histological Examination

All rats were sacrificed after feeding for 26 weeks. Their esophagi, stomachs, small intestines, and large intestines were removed and dissected longitudinally. The location, shape, size, and number of tumors generated were recorded. All tumors were then fixed with 10% formalin for histological examination.

5. Statistical Analysis

The significance of differences in tumor incidence was analyzed using the x^2 test, and the remaining data were analyzed by Student's t-test.

B. RESULTS
1. Body Weights

During the experiment, body weights of rats treated with AOM were generally lower than those without AOM treatment. In most cases, however, the differences were not statistically significant. Statistical differences of body weight were observed between the following groups: AOM-treated and untreated on week 9 ($p<0.05$) and AOM-control and AOM-GTP2 on weeks 13, 17, and 21 ($p<0.05$, $p<0.005$, and $p<0.05$), respectively. At autopsy on week 26, the body weights among the six reference groups were not significantly different (Figure 3).

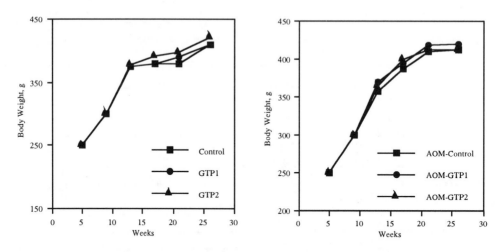

Figure 3. Body weights during the experiment. Reproduced from Yamane et al. (1991) [25] by permission of Japan Cancer Association, Tokyo.

2. Colon Tumors

Histologically, the colon tumors consisted of atypical glands, and basophilically stained cells with large number of mitotic bodies were often observed. The nuclei were large and were located at different sites in the cytoplasm. Tumor cells often invaded submucosal space, proper muscle layer, and subserosal space.

3. Inhibition by GTP

Rats without the AOM treatment (i.e., control, GTP1, and GTP2) had no colon tumors. The inhibitory effect of GTP on AOM-induced colon tumors is summarized in Table 2. The percent of rats bearing tumors in the AOM-control group was 77%. On the other hand, the percent of those in the AOM-GTP1 and AOM-GTP2 groups was 38% ($p<0.005$) and 48% ($p<0.05$), respectively. The difference between the AOM-GTP1 and the AOM-GTP2 groups was not statistically significant. The average number of tumors per rat in the AOM-control group was 1.5, whereas those of the AOM-GTP1 and AOM-GTP2 groups were only 0.6 ($p<0.01$) and 0.7 ($p<0.01$), respectively. The mean tumor diameter among the three AOM-treated groups was not significantly different. The average distance of colon tumors from the anus was 10.5±5.5 cm (mean ±S.D.) for AOM-control, 7.1±3.9 cm for AOM-GTP1, and 10.4±5.4 cm for AOM-GTP2, which were not significantly different.

V. CONCLUSIONS

Based on various data obtained by many epidemiological studies carried out in numerous laboratories, it is highly possible to conclude that green tea

Table 2
Inhibitory Effect of Green Tea Polyphenols on AOM-Induced Colon Carcinogenesis

Treatment Group	Tumor Incidence Ratio[1]	Total Number of Tumors	Tumors per Rat[2]	Diameter of Tumors (mm)[3]
AOM-Control	17/22 (77)	33	1.5 ± 0.2	5.6 ± 3.4
AOM-GTP1	8/21 (38)**	13	0.6 ± 0.2***	5.4 ± 2.8
AOM-GTP2	10/21 (48)*	14	0.7 ± 0.2***	6.4 ± 3.0

[1]Numbers in parentheses are the percent of rats bearing tumors.
[2]Mean ±S.E.   [3]Mean ±S.D.
Significant difference from the AOM-control group: *, $p<0.05$; **, $p<0.005$; ***, $p<0.01$.
Reproduced from Yamane et al. (1991) [25] by permission of Japan Cancer Association, Tokyo.

shows beneficial effects to reduce cancer risk. Also, it is clear that epigallocatechin gallate, which is the major constituent of the green tea polyphenols examined, is the compound responsible for bringing on the cancer preventive effect on cancer.

For elucidation of the mechanism involved in the effect of tea polyphenols to interfere with the initiation, growth, and subsequent progression of specific cancers, further study will be necessary. The study, of course, provides a general concept about the relation between tea polyphenols and human health. Regarding this, biochemical mechanisms for the inhibition of tumorigenesis by tea polyphenols have been emphasized by the results of various experiments. The chemical and biochemical functions of green tea polyphenols proposed are summarized as follows:

a. Antioxidative activities of green tea polyphenols

Green tea polyphenols are strong scavengers for oxidative radicals that bring damage to DNA. Also, catechin moiety of tea polyphenols is a strong metal ion chelator. It can bind and decrease the level of ferric ions which are required for generation of reactive oxygen radicals by Fenton-type reaction.

b. Trapping of carcinogens

The structure of tea polyphenols possesses strong nucleophilic centers at positions C-6 and C-8. This property provides an opportunity to react with electrophilic carcinogenic species to form a tea polyphenol-carcinogen adduct that may result in the prevention of tumorigenesis.

c. Inhibition of nitrosation reactions

N-nitroso compounds are known to be implicated in etiologic factors of gastric, esophageal, and other cancers. Tea polyphenols have been demonstrated to react with nitrosating species and thus, inhibit nitrosation. This property is important to suppressively affect cancers caused by endogenously formed N-nitroso compounds.

d. Inhibition of the growth of intestinal clostridia

It was suggested that tumor growth or malignant transformation is correlated with the increase of certain *Clostridium* genera bacteria. The bacteria have been reported to participate in the biotransformation of a variety of ingested or endogenously formed compounds to carcinogenic products such as nitroso-compounds and aromatic steroids. Tea polyphenols inhibit the growth of clostridia selectively among various intestinal bacteria. This effect of tea polyphenols may also explain the important role in inhibition of the AOM-induced colon carcinogenesis.

e. Inhibition of biochemical signals of tumor initiation

Cytochrome P-450 is the major enzyme responsible for production of procarcinogen metabolites which bind DNA. This binding to DNA is essential for tumor initiation. Tea polyphenols inhibit P-450-dependent arylhydrocarbon hydroxylase, 7-ethoxycoumari-*O*-deethylase, and 7-ethoxyresorsi-*N*-*O*-deethylase activities. The ability to inhibit the key determinant enzymatic pathways for cancer initiation would be expected to have favorable protection against carcinogenesis.

f. Inhibition of biochemical signals of tumor promotion

The induction of ornithine decarboxylase (ODC) and protein kinase C activities by phorbol esters, e.g. TPA, is closely related to the tumor-promoting activity shown by a variety of tumor promoters. Topical application of tea polyphenols to mouse skin was found to inhibit TPA-mediated induction of epidermal ODC activities in a dose dependent way.

The mechanisms proposed above are thought to affect carcinogenesis by single or combinational mechanisms, and they might contribute to the overall protective effect of green tea against cancer. On the other hand, it has been recognized that heterocyclic amines (HCA) which are formed during the cooking of meats and fish are genotoxic carcinogens associated with the principal types of cancer found in meat-eating people such as breast, colon, or pancreas cancers. Recently, tea polyphenols were found to prevent the formation of heterocyclic amine by competitively trapping the Maillard reaction intermediates which lead to HCA [26]. This novel finding that tea polyphenols block the formation of HCA while cooking meat and fish may give alternative procedures for minimizing cancer risk. Tea has a long history as a popular beverage without any harmful effect, such as the mutagenecity showed by coffee [27], so that it can safely be applied clinically for cancer prevention. Therefore, studies on the biochemical and physiological fate of tea polyphenols in our body will be a particularly important subject to be solved in detail. In this regard, recently a remarkable result has been reported by Lee's group in the U.S.A. [28]. They have developed the methodology for analysis of tea polyphenols in human plasma and urine, using HPLC with the coulochem electrode array detection system. For example, plasma samples were collected from the volunteers one hour after drinking 1.2 g of green tea extract which contained 46-258 ng/ml of EGCg, 82-206 ng/ml of EGC, and 48-80 ng/ml of EC, and they were analyzed. The result demonstrated the evidence of the absorption of tea polyphenol and also suggested that they might function as useful markers for quantifying human ingestion of tea. In addition, a similar experiment using rats has been carried out by Japanese researchers [29]. Male Wister rats were administered orally with 50 mg of EGCg, and the plasma of rats was evaluated by using HPLC equipped with electrochemical detector (ECD). EGCg was detected in the rat plasma after oral administration, and time-course of plasma EGCg showed that the highest level of EGCg was observed about one hour later in the experimental period. These results are a step forward for studying the effect of tea consumption on human cancers.

REFERENCES

1. **Agarwal, R. and Mukhtar, H.,** Cutaneous chemical carcinogenesis, in *Pharmacology of the Skin*, Mukhtar, H., Ed., CRC Press, Boca Raton, Florida, 1991, p 371.
2. **Greenwald, P.,** Micronutrients and chemoprevention, in *Cancer: Principles and practice of oncology*, De-Vita, V. T., Hellman, S., and Rosenberg, S. A., Eds., J. B. Lippincott, Philadelphia, 1993, p 457.
3. **Oguni, I., Chen, S. J., Lin, P. Z., and Hara, Y.,** Protection against cancer risk by Japanese green tea, *Prev. Med.*, **21**, 332, 1992.
4. **WHO,** International agency for research on cancer: coffee, tea mate, methylxanthines and methylglyoxal, *IARC Mongor. Eval. Carcinog. Risk Hum.*, Lyom. IARC Press, 1991, p 207.
5. **Yang, C. S. and Wang, Z.-Y.,** Tea and cancer, *Journal of the National Cancer Institute*, **85**, 1038, 1993.
6. **Kaufman, B. D., Liberman, I. S., and Tyshetsky, V. I.,** Some data concerning the incidence of oesohageal cancer in the Gurjev region of the Kazakh SSR (Russ.), *Vopr. Onkol.*, **11**, 78, 1965.
7. **Kono, S., Ikeda, M., Tokudome, S., and Kuratune, M.,** A case-control study of gastric cancer and diet in northern Kyushu, Japan, *Jpn. J. Cancer Res.*, **79**, 1067, 1988.
8. **Shim, J. S., Kang, M. H., Kim, Y. H., Roh, J. K., Roberts, C., and Lee, I. P.,** Chemopreventive effect of green tea (*Camellia sinensis*) among cigarette smokers, *Cancer Epidemiol. Biomarkers & Prev.*, **4**, 387, 1995.
9. **Han, C. and Xu, Y.,** The effect of Chinese tea on the occurrence of esophageal tumor induced by N- nitrosomethylbenzylamine in rats, *Biomed. Environ. Sci.*, **3**, 35, 1990.
10. **Wang, Z. Y., Agarwal, R., Khan, W. A., and Mukhtar, H.,** Protection against benzo(*a*)pyrene and N-nitrosodiethylamine-induced lung and forestomach tumorigenesis in A/J mice by water extracts of green tea and licorice, *Carcinogenesis*, **13**, 1491, 1992.
11. **Yaname, T., Takahashi, T., Kuwata, K., Oya, K., Inagake, M., Kitao, Y., Suganuma, M., and Fujiki, H.,** Inhibition of N-methyl-N'-nitro-N-nitrosoguanidine-induced carcinogenesis by (-)-epigallocatechin gallate in the rat glandular stomach, *Cancer Res.*, **55**, 2081, 1995.

12. **Fujita, Y., Yamane, T., Tanaka, M., Kuwata, K., Okuzumi, J., Takahashi, T., Fujiki, H., and Okuda, T.**, Inhibitory effect of (-)-epigallocatechin gallate on carcinogenesis with N-ethyl-N'-nitro-N-nitrosoguanidine in mouse duodenum, *Jpn. J. Cancer Res.*, **80**, 503, 1989.
13. **Wang, Z. Y., Agarwal, R., Bickers, D. R., and Mukhtar, H.**, Protection against ultraviolet B radiation-induced photocarcinogenesis in hairless mice by green tea polyphenols, *Carcinogenesis*, **12**, 1527, 1991.
14. **Khan, W. A., Wang, Z. Y., Athar, M., Bickers, D. R., and Mukhtar, H.**, Inhibition of the skin tumorigenecity of (+) 7β, 8α-dihydroxy-9α, 10α-epoxy-7, 8, 9, 10-tetrahydrobenzo (a)pyrene by tannic acid, green tea polyphenols and quercetin in Sencar mice, *Cancer Lett.*, **42**, 7, 1988.
15. **Katiyar, S. K., Agarwal, R., Wang, Z. Y., Bhatia, A. K., and Mukhtar, H.**, (-)-Epigallocatechin-3-gallate in *Camellia sinensis* leaves from Himalayan region of Sikkim: inhibitory effects against biochemical events and tumor initiation in Sencar mouse skin, *Nutr. Cancer*, **18**, 73, 1992.
16. **Wang, Z. Y., Huang, M. T., Ferraro, T., Wong, C. Q., Lou, Y. R., Reuhl, K., Latropoulos, M., Yang, C. S., and Conney, A. H.**, Inhibitory effect of green tea in the drinking water on tumorigenesis by ultraviolet light and 12-O-tetradecanoylphorbol-13-acetate in the skin of SKH-1 mice, *Cancer Res.*, **52**, 1162, 1992.
17. **Wang, Z. Y., Hong, J.-Y., Huang, M.-T., Reuhl, K. R., Conney, A. H., and Yang, C. S.**, Inhibition of N-nitrosodiethylamine- and 4-(methylnitrosamino)-1(3-pyridyl)-1-butanone-induced tumorigenesis in A/J mice by green tea and black tea, *Cancer Res.*, **52**, 1943, 1992.
18. **Xu, Y., Ho, C. T., Amin, S. G., Han, C., and Chung, F. L.**, Inhibition of tobacco-specific nitrosamine-induced lung tumorigenesis in A/J mice by green tea and its major polyphenol as antioxidants, *Cancer Res.*, **52**, 3875, 1992.
19. **Masuda, M., Takasuka, N., Murakoshi, M., Baba, M., Onozuka, M., Sugimoto, H., Satomi, Y., Kim, M., and Nishino, H.**, Preventive effect of oral administration of green tea polyphenols on lung tumorigenesis in mice, *Proceedings of the Japanese Cancer Association*, 134, 1995.
20. **Li, Y.**, Comparative study on the inhibitory effect of green tea, coffee and levamisole on the hepatocarcinogenic action of diethylnitrosamine, *Chung Hua Chung Liu Tsa Chih (Chinese J. Cancer)*, **13**, 193, 1991.
21. **Harada, N., Takabayashi, F., Oguni, I., and Hara, Y.**, Anti-promotion effect of green tea extracts on pancreatic cancer in golden hamster induced by N-nitroso-bis (2-oxopropyl) amine, in *Proceedings of the International Symposium on Tea Science,* Kurofune Printing Co. Ltd., Shizuoka, 1991, p 200.
22. **Hara, Y.**, Prophylactic function of tea polyphenols, *The 204th American Chemical Society National Meeting in Washington, D.C.,* 1992.
23. **Ahn, Y. J., Kawamura, T., Kim, M., Yamamoto, T., and Mitsuoka, T.**, Tea polyphenols: selective growth inhibitors of *Clostridium* spp., *Agric. Biol. Chem.*, **55**, 1425, 1991.
24. **Okubo, T., Ishihara, N., Oura, A., Serit, M., Kim, M., Yamamoto, T., and Mitsuoka, T.**, *In vivo* effects of tea polyphenol intake on human intestinal microflora and metabolism, *Biosci. Biotech. Biochem.*, **56**, 588, 1992.

25. **Yamane, T., Hagiwara, N., Tateishi, M., Akachi, S., Kim, M., Okuzumi, J., Kitao, Y., Inagake, M., Kuwata, K., and Takahashi, T.,** Inhibition of azoxymethane-induced colon carcinogenesis in rat by green tea polyphenol fraction, *Jpn. J. Cancer Res.*, **82**, 1336, 1991.
26. **Weisburger, J. H., Nagao, M., Wakabayashi, K., and Oguri, A.,** Prevention of heterocyclic amine formation by tea and tea polyphenols, *Cancer Lett.*, **83**, 143, 1994.
27. **Mure, K., Takeuchi, T., Takeshita, T., and Morimoto, K.,** Genotoxic Potentials of Life styles (6) Assessment of Chromosome alteration (Micronucleus) and Urinary Mutagenicity, *Proceedings of the Japanese Cancer Association*, 705, 1995.
28. **Lee, M.-J., Wang, Z.-Y., Li, H., Chen, L., Sun, Y., Gobbo, S., Balentine, D. A., and Yang, C. S.,** Analysis of plasma and urinary tea polyphenols in human subjects, *Cancer Epidemiol. Biomarkers & Prev.*, **4**, 393, 1995.
29. **Unno, T. and Takeo, T.,** Absorption of (-)-epigallocatechin gallate into the circulation system of rats, *Biosci. Biotech. Biochem.*, **59**, 1558, 1995.

Chapter 7

SUPPRESSIVE EFFECT OF UREMIC TOXIN FORMATION BY TEA POLYPHENOLS

S. Sakanaka and M. Kim

TABLE OF CONTENTS

I. Introduction
II. Renal Failure and Uremic Toxin
    A. Animal Model of Adenine-Induced Chronic Renal Failure
    B. Methylguanidine as Uremic Toxin
III. Effect of Tea Polyphenols on Urinary Methylguanidine Excretion
IV. Decrease in Uremic Toxin Production by Tea Polyphenols in Humans
    Acknowledgments
    References

I. INTRODUCTION

It has been shown by various recent studies that active oxygen species (free radicals) produced in organ tissue are concerned with the cause of various diseases such as inflammation, cancer, abnormal aging, etc. Renal failure is also thought to be one of these diseases. We have the mechanisms of controlling the active oxygen species or free radicals by means of enzymic level, such as superoxide dismutase, catalase, peroxidase, or various antioxidants such as transferrin, glutathione, ascorbic acid, tocopherols, and so on (Table 1). However, it is likely that hydroxyl ($\cdot OH$) radicals are not controlled completely by the enzymes or biochemicals above [1].

It is known that hydroxyl radicals among active oxygen species are most closely related to the injury of organ tissue. Hydroxyl radicals are produced from $^-O_2$ and H_2O_2, and the rate of these reactions is stimulated to become faster in the presence of small amounts of chelated ferric iron. Hydroxyl radicals are also produced from H_2O by the radial rays. Hydroxyl radicals have very high reactivity but short-lived compared with other active oxygen species. Since there is no system to eliminate hydroxyl radicals in our organ tissues, the radicals are thought to be highly dangerous to various tissue.

The kidneys are indispensable organs for the excretion of waste metabolites and various other unnecessary substances from body. A decrease in the function of the kidneys causes accumulation of uremic toxin, and as a result the symptoms of uremia occur. This is the so-called renal failure. The patients with renal failure are generally subjected to a high oxidative stress state [2-5]. Methylguanidine, a uremic toxin, is derived from creatinine by the action of active oxygen, especially by the hydroxyl radicals [6-10], and it has been suggested that the active oxygen causes occurrence of renal failure. This chapter describes the effect of green tea polyphenols on hydroxyl radicals, demonstrating that green tea polyphenols suppress the production of uremic toxin (methylguanidine) and thus, improve the renal failure observed in human volunteers.

Table 1
Antioxidative Biological Systems

Antioxidant	Function
Preventive antioxidant	
Glutathione peroxidase	$H_2O_2 + 2\,GSH \longrightarrow 2\,H_2O + GSSG$
	$LOOH + 2\,GSH \longrightarrow LOH + H_2O + GSSG$
Catalase	$2H_2O_2 \longrightarrow 2H_2O + O$
Peroxidase	$H_2O_2 + AH \longrightarrow 2H_2O + A$
Transferrin	⎱
Ferritin	chelated iron
Lactoferrin	⎰
Ceruloplasmin	chelated copper
β-Carotene	quenched singlet oxygen
Superoxide dismutase (SOD)	$2O_2^- + 2H^+ \longrightarrow H_2O_2 + O_2$
Chain-breaking antioxidant	
Vitamin C	
Uric acid	
Bilirubin	scavenging oxygen radicals and breaking chain sequence
Ubiquinol	
Vitamin E	

II. RENAL FAILURE AND UREMIC TOXIN

A. ANIMAL MODELS OF ADENINE-INDUCED CHRONIC RENAL FAILURE

Yokozawa and her coworkers have established a method of rat models for experimental chronic renal failure by oral administration of adenine. They also confirmed that this rat model suffers from true uremia histologically and biochemically [11-13]. Macroscopically, the kidneys were enlarged and colored in pale gray by the administration of a 0.75% adenine diet (Figure 1).

Renal histological analysis revealed that many needle crystals with positive polarization in the renal tubular lumina and interstitium appeared. A compound of the crystals was identified to be 2, 8-dihydroxyadenine. In addition to the changes in urea nitrogen, creatinine, and uric acid, several other abnormal symptoms were observed. A marked elevation of allantoin, increase in methylguanidine and guanidinosuccinic acid, abnormal blood and urinary amino acid patterns, abnormal electrolyte metabolism, and polyuria.

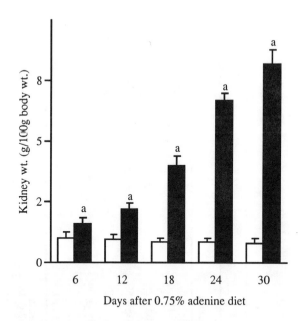

Figure 1. Kidney weight of rats fed on 0.75% adenine diet.
Values are mean ± S.E. of 6 rats. [a] Significantly different from the value of rats fed on the control diet, $p<0.001$. □, control diet ; ■, 0.75% adenine diet. Reproduced from Yokozawa et al. (1982) [11] by permission of the Japan Society for Bioscience, Biotechnology, and Agrochemistry, Tokyo.

B. METHYLGUANIDINE AS UREMIC TOXIN

Uremic toxin is a substance which accumulates in the organ tissue as renal failure progresses, causing several specific symptoms of uremia.

Methylguanidine is the most relevant toxin to uremia among various uremic toxins including guanidinosuccinic acid, dimethylamine, myoinositol, etc. Methylguanidine has also been reported to be an inhibitor of ATPase, oxidative phosphorylation, lactate dehydrogenase, and certain platelet factors [14-17]. Methylguanidine, on one hand, has been found to accumulate in the organ tissue as the excretional function of the kidney declines.

It has been reported that methylguanidine is produced from creatol (5-hydroxycreatinine), an intermediary product in the metabolism of creatinine by the reaction with hydroxyl radicals (Figure 2). The estimation of the hydroxyl radicals has thus been achieved by the indirect method of determining methylguanidine produced [6-10]. In the case of renal failure, active oxygen increases in quantity and reacts with creatinine to result in enhanced production of methylguanidine (Table 2) [18].

In addition, due to accumulation in organ tissue, methylguanidine is considered difficult to be removed by hemodialysis. Therefore, methylguanidine has been thought to be involved in various uremia-like symptoms as a causative toxic agent.

Table 2
Methylguanidine Production in Normal Rats and Renal Failure Rats (μg/100 g body weight)

	Normal			Renal failure		
	Cr(−)	Cr(+)	Cr(+)−Cr(−)	Cr(−)	Cr(+)	Cr(+)−Cr(−)
Serum	n.d.	n.d.	0	0.53±0.16	3.82±0.37**	3.29
Liver	n.d.	0.08±0.03**	0.08	0.96±0.26	4.72±0.36**	3.76
Kidney	0.01±0.01	0.01±0.06*	0.10	2.03±0.59	10.54±0.69**	8.51
Muscle	6.35±0.19	7.85±0.76*	1.50	29.42±8.29	150.06±9.82	120.64
Urine	1.09±0.21	69.71±4.23**	68.62	14.97±4.98	50.86±8.15	35.89
Total	7.45±0.28	77.75±4.30**	70.30	47.91±10.44	220.00±12.75**	172.09

Cr(−), before creatinine administration; Cr(+), after creatinine administration; n.d., not detectable.
Significance of differences from the value of rats before creatinine administration: *, $p<0.05$; **, $p<0.001$.
Reproduced from Yokozawa et al. (1990) [18] by permission of S. Karger AG, Basel.

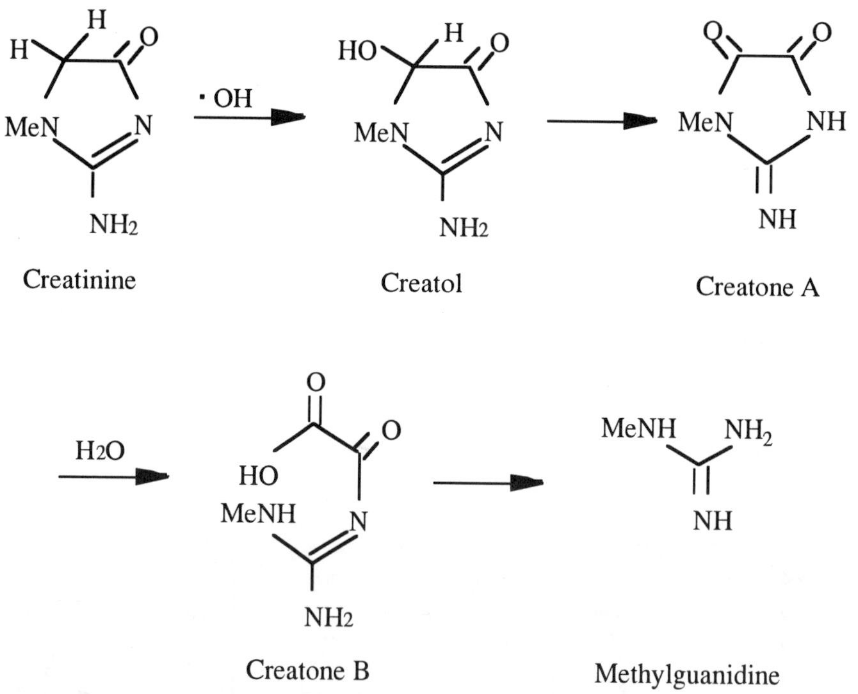

Figure 2. Formation of methylguanidine.

III. EFFECT OF TEA POLYPHENOLS ON URINARY METHYLGUANIDINE EXCRETION

The hydroxyl radical scavenging reaction of green tea polyphenols was examined in rats with experimental renal failure induced by adenine administration [19]. Methylguanidine accumulated in the organ tissue in parallel with the progress of renal failure after adenine administration. The degree of scavenging reaction was estimated by the urinary methylguanidine excretion as an index.

The LWH Wistar rats were fed *ad libitum* on an 18% casein diet containing 0.75% adenine for 24 days and the casein diet without adenine for a subsequent 10 days to produce experimental renal failure in the animals. The renal failure was observed after 6 days of adenine administration. The tea polyphenols used here were composed of (-)-epigallocatechin gallate (18%), (-)-gallocatechin gallate (11.6%), (-)-epicatechin gallate (4.6%), (-)-epigallocatechin (15.0%), (+)-gallocatechin (14.8%), (-)-epicatechin (7.0%), (+)-catechin (3.5%). In addition to this rat group, the experiment of using (-)-epigallocatechin gallate alone was also carried out. The green tea polyphenols or (-)-epigallocatechin gallate were dissolved in water and given orally as drinking water for 14 days after the adenine administration for 20 days. Control rats were given the corresponding volume of water alone. Each rat was separately fed in a metabolic cage, and a 24 h urine sample was collected everyday during the 20th to 34th days of the experiment.

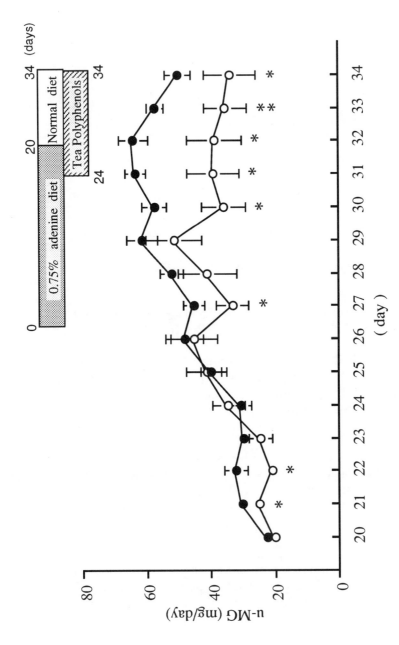

Figure 3. Effect of tea polyphenols on urinary methylguanidine (u-MG) excretion.
—●—, control group; —○—, tea polyphenols treated-group (2 mg/rat/day); *, p<0.05; **, p<0.01. Reproduced from Yokozawa et al. (1992) [19] by permission of the Japan Society for Bioscience, Biotechnology, and Agrochemistry, Tokyo.

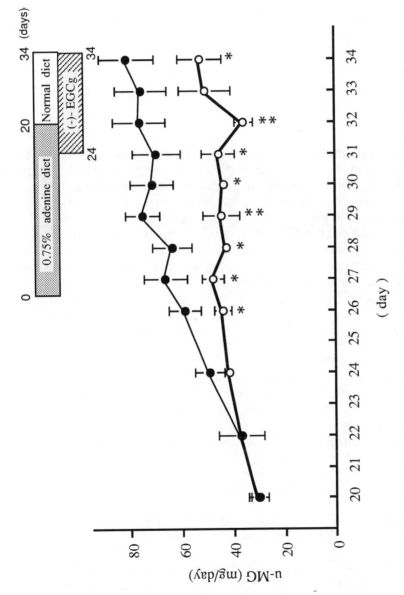

Figure 4. Effect of (-)-epigallocatechin gallate (EGCg) on urinary methylguanidine (u-MG) excretion. ●, control group; ○, (-)-epigallocatechin gallate treated-group (0.5 mg/rat/day); *, $p<0.05$; **, $p<0.01$. Reproduced from Yokozawa et al. (1992) [19] by permission of the Japan Society for Bioscience, Biotechnology, and Agrochemistry, Tokyo.

Table 3
Effect of (-)-Epicatechin 3-O-gallate on Serum Constituents

Group	Dose mg/kg BW/day	Urea nitrogen mg/dl	Creatinine mg/dl	Methylguanidine µg/dl
Control	-	125.1±12.4	3.64±0.15	11.19±1.39
(-)-Epicatechin 3-O-gallate	2.5	95.7±6.7*	3.25±0.18	7.03±0.85*
(-)-Epicatechin 3-O-gallate	5	90.8±5.3*	3.06±0.10**	7.40±0.68*
(-)-Epicatechin 3-O-gallate	10	91.2±2.9*	2.92±0.19**	8.12±0.89*

*, $p<0.05$; **, $p<0.01$, i.e., significantly different from control value.
Reproduced from Yokozawa et al. (1991) [20] by permission of S. Karger AG, Basel.

Methylguanidine in deproteinized urine was separated by HPLC using a strong acid cation-exchanger and quantified by the fluorescence development (excitation, 365 nm; emission, 495 nm). Changes in urinary methylguanidine of the green tea polyphenols treated and control rats under the experimental conditions are shown in Figure 3. Rats given 0.5 mg green tea polyphenols per day showed almost a constant excretion of urinary methylguanidine throughout the experimental period. The excretion from rats given 1 mg green tea polyphenols per day tended to decrease from the 21st day in comparison with the control rats and significantly decreased on the 30th day. In rats given 2 mg green tea polyphenols per day, the urinary methylguanidine excretion was significantly lower than the controls, and this phenomenon continued until the 34th day. The degree of decrease in methylgunidine excretion was 16-40% of that of the controls. Figure 4 shows the effect of (-) epigallocatechin gallate on the urinary methylguanidine excretion. In the rats given 0.5 mg (-)-epigallocatechin gallate, the urinary methylguanidine excretion markedly decreased from the 6th day to the end of the experiment, indicating that the effect of (-)-epigallocatechin gallate was greater than that of the green tea polyphenols at the same dose.

It has already been reported that a decrease in the urinary methylguanidine excretion is resulted by (-)-epicatechin 3-O-gallate (Table 3) [20] and by (+)-catechin [21]. Taking these findings into consideration, it may be concluded that green tea polyphenols exhibit a radical scavenging action.

IV. DECREASE IN UREMIC TOXIN PRODUCTION BY TEA POLYPHENOLS IN HUMANS

Recently, it has been reported that the injury by amidosis is due to active oxygen and thus, the free radical activity of hemodialysis patients has been studied. Methylguanidine is known to be a causal toxin of such diseases as anorexia, gastric ulcer, neuropathy, and anemia [22]. As described above, the production of methylguanidine is considered to be attributed mainly to hydroxyl radicals. Renal failure patients, therefore, seem to suffer from a high oxidative stress by the increase in the formation of active oxygen or by the decrease in elimination activity of active oxygen.

The clinical efficacy of green tea polyphenols for suppression of the formation of methylguanidine was investigated [23]. Fifty volunteers who were hemodialysis patients were administrated with two jellies per day for 6 months. Each jelly contained 200 mg of green tea polyphenols. Volunteers' serum methylguanidine contents were measured every month. Methylguanidine content decreased significantly in one month after the administration of green tea polyphenols (Figure 5). In 6 months after the administration, the mean content of methylguanidine was about 70% of that at the beginning of the treatment. The decreasing rate was greater in the high content group than the low content group of methylguanidine. The ratio of methylguanidine to creatinine was also decreased by administration of green tea polyphenols. Nevertheless, the production of methylguanidine was not necessarily related with the content of creatinine (Figure 6). The experiment above is evidence that the application of tea polyphenols results in suppression of methylguanidine production in hemodialysis patients as a result of their radical scavenger action on the hydroxyl radicals.

The study of methylguanidine production in organ tissue as an index of oxidative radical formation has suggested that green tea polyphenols induce the recovery from oxidative stress. This idea may open a novel application for green tea polyphenols as a material for prevention and therapy of oxidative stress diseases.

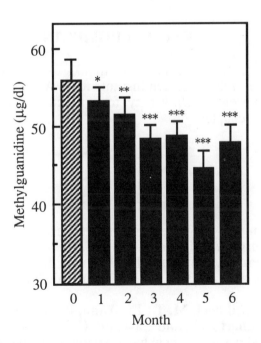

Figure 5. Effect of tea polyphenols on contents of serum methylguanidine. (n=50) *, $p<0.05$; **, $p<0.01$; ***, $p<0.001$.

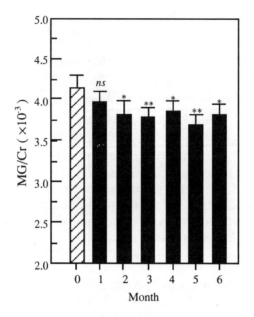

Figure 6. Effect of tea polyphenols on serum MG/Cr ratio (n=50). *, $p<0.05$; **, $p<0.01$; ns, not significant.

ACKNOWLEDGMENTS

The authors wish to express sincere thanks to Dr. Takako Yokozawa, Associate Professor of the Research Institute for WAKAN-YAKU of Toyama Medical and Pharmaceutical University, for her kind discussion, useful advice, and revision of this chapter.

REFERENCES

1. **Niki, E.,** Vitamine E and its related compounds as antioxidants, *Yuki Gosei Kagaku Kyokaishi (in Japanese),* **47**, 902, 1989.
2. **Fillit, H., Elion, E., Sullivan, J., Sherman, R., and Zabriskie, J. B.,** Thiobarbituric acid reactive material in uremic blood, *Nephron,* **29**, 40, 1981.
3. **Giardini, O., Gallucci, M. T., Lubrano, R., Tenore, G. R., Bandino, D., Silvi, I., Ruberto, U., and Casciani, C. I.,** Evidence of red blood cell membrane lipid peroxidation in haemodialysis patients, *Nephron,* **36**, 235, 1984.
4. **Kuroda, M., Asaka, B., Tofuku, Y., and Takeda, R.,** Serum antioxidant activity in uremic patients, *Nephron,* **41**, 293, 1985.
5. **Flament, J., Goldman, M., Waterlot, Y., Dupont, E., Wybran, J., and**

Vanherweghem, J. L., Impairment of phagocyte oxidative metabolism in hemodialyzed patients with iron overload, *Clin. Nephrol.*, **25**, 227, 1986.
6. **Nakamura, K., Ienaga, K., Yokozawa, M., Fujituka, N., and Oura, H.,** Production of methylguanidine from creatinine via creatol by active oxygen species: analysis of the catabolism *in vitro, Nephron,* **58**, 42, 1991.
7. **Yokozawa, T., Fujituka, N., Oura, H., Ienaga, K., and Nakamura, K.,** Comparison of methylguanidine production from creatinine and creatol *in vivo, Nephron,* **58**, 125, 1991.
8. **Ienaga, K., Nakamura, K., Yamakawa, M., Toyomaki, Y., Matuura, H., Yokozawa, T., Oura, H., and Nakano, K.,** The use of ^{13}C-labelling to prove that creatinine is oxidized by mammal into creatol and 5-hydroxy-1-methylhydantoin, *J. Chem. Soc. Chem. Commun.*, 509, 1991.
9. **Yokozawa, T., Fujituka, N., and Oura, H.,** Contribution of hydroxyl radical to the production of methylguanidine from creatinine, *Nephron,* **59**, 662, 1991.
10. **Yokozawa, T., Fujituka, N., Oura, H., and Hattori, M.,** Contribution of active oxygen to the production of methylguanidine using alloxan, *Nephron,* **60**, 369, 1992.
11. **Yokozawa, T., Oura, H., Nakagawa, H., and Okada, T.,** Adenine-induced hyperuricemia and renal damage in rats, *Nippon Nogeikagaku Kaishi (in Japanese)*, **56**, 655, 1982.
12. **Yokozawa, T., Zheng, P. D., Oura, H., and Koizumi, F.,** Animal model of adenine-induced chronic renal failure in rats, *Nephron,* **44**, 230, 1986.
13. **Yokozawa, T., Chung, H. Y., and Oura, H.,** Urinary constituents and renal function in rats administered with adenine, *Jap. J. Nephrol.,* **29**, 1129, 1987.
14. **Giovannetti, B., Cioni, L., Balestri, P. L., and Biagini, M.,** Evidence that guanidines and some related compounds cause haemolysis in chronic uraemia, *Clin. Sci.,* **34**, 141, 1968.
15. **Rajagopalan, K. V., Fridovich, I., and Handler, P.,** Inhibition of enzyme activity by urea, *Fed. Proc.,* **19**, 49, 1960.
16. **Hollunger, G.,** Guanidines and oxidative phosphorylation, *Acta Pharmacol.,* **11**, 7, 1955.
17. **Cahalane, B. F., Johnson, B. A., Monto, R. W., and Galdwell, M. J.,** Acquired thrombocytopathy: observations on the coagulation defect in uremia, *Am. J. Clin. Path.,* **30**, 507, 1958.
18. **Yokozawa, T., Fujitsuka, N., and Oura, H.,** Production of methylguanidine from creatinine in normal rats and rats with renal failure, *Nephron,* **56**, 249, 1990.
19. **Yokozawa, T., Oura, H., Sakanaka, S., and Kim, M.,** Effect of tannins in green tea on the urinary methylguanidine excretion in rats indicating a possible radical scavenging action, *Biosci. Biotech. Biochem.,* **56**, 896, 1992.
20. **Yokozawa, T., Fujioka, K., Oura, H., Nonaka, G., and Nishioka, I.,** Effects of rhubarb tannins on uremic toxins, *Nephron,* **58**, 155, 1991.
21. **Fujioka, K., Yokozawa, T., Oura, H., Hattori, M., Nonaka, G., and Nishioka, I.,** in *The 8th General Meeting of Medical and Pharmaceutical Society for WAKAN-YAKU in Osaka*, Japan, 1991, 66.

22. **Giovannetti, B., Biagini, M., Balestri, P. L., Navalesi, R., Giagnoni, P., de Matteis, A., Ferro-Milone, P., and Perfetti, C.,** Uremia-like syndrome in dogs chronically intoxicated with methylguanidine and creatinine, *Clin. Sci.*, **36**, 445, 1969.
23. **Yokozawa, T., Oura, H., Shibata, T., Ishida, K., Kaneko, M., Hasegawa, M., Sakanaka, S., and Kim, M.,** Effect of green tea tannin in dialysis patients, *J. Trad. Med.*, **13**, 124, 1996.

Chapter 8

GREEN TEA POLYPHENOLS FOR PREVENTION OF DENTAL CARIES

S. Sakanaka

TABLE OF CONTENTS

I. Introduction
II. Dental Diseases
III. Effects of Tea Polyphenols on Cariogenicity Observed in *In Vitro* Tests
    A. Components of Tea Polyphenols and Their Effects on Growth of Cariogenic Bacteria
        1. Components of Tea Polyphenols
        2. Inhibitory Activities of Polyphenol Compounds
    B. Inhibitory Effects of Tea Polyphenols on Enzymic Synthesis of Glucans and Adherence of Bacterial Cells on Tooth Surface
IV. Effects of Tea Polyphenols on Dental Caries and Plaques
    A. Effects of Tea Polyphenols on Dental Carries in Rats
    B. Effects of Tea Polyphenols on Plaque Formation in Men
    C. Epidemiological Survey of the Effect of Green Tea Drinking for Dental Caries Risk in Men
V. Recent Trends and Future Aspects of the Application of Green Tea Polyphenols
References

I. INTRODUCTION

The infusion of dried tea leaves is one of the most popular beverages in the world. The tea plant is cultivated widely from tropical to temperate zones of the world. There are many types and grades of tea available in the market, but they are classified principally into green tea, oolong tea, and black tea [1, 2]. In Japan, the infusion of green tea (non-fermented tea) is often taken few times a day, especially after meals. There is a traditional saying that "drinking green tea makes our mouth clean." About thirty years ago, a research group suggested green tea infusion efficacy for prevention of dental caries, because tea leaves contain a considerably high concentration of fluorides [3]. The research group observed that tea drinking only once after school lunch resulted in a decrease of the risk of dental caries in children [4]. However, they could not attribute this result to the action of fluoride alone, because it was shown that tea extract was much more effective in the preventive effect than fluoride of the same concentration [5].

We investigated the green tea components which affected the cariogenic bacteria and found that several tea polyphenols are effective in preventing the dental caries [6-8]. In this chapter, isolation of the active polyphenols from green tea leaves extract and their preventive effects on dental caries evidenced in both *in vitro* and *in vivo* tests are described.

II. DENTAL DISEASES

Dental caries and periodontal diseases are the main infectious diseases of our oral cavity. These diseases are induced by oral microflora. Among hundreds of microorganisms indigenous to the oral cavity, only cariogenic streptococci, especially *Streptococcus mutans*, play a key role in the cause of dental caries [9].

Figure 1 shows the mechanism of dental caries. *S. mutans* synthesizes water-insoluble glucan from sucrose in foods and drinks. *S. mutans* and other microorganisms grow in the synthesized polysaccharides (glucans) called dental plaque. The bacteria grown there, metabolize various saccharides and produce organic acids, especially lactic acid which is retained in dental plaque eventually to decalcify the tooth enamel. Usually one cannot recognize dental caries before it gets worse to a considerable extent. The tooth surface once plagued, is never brought back to the original state. Therefore, prevention of dental caries is much more important than the cure of the plagued teeth.

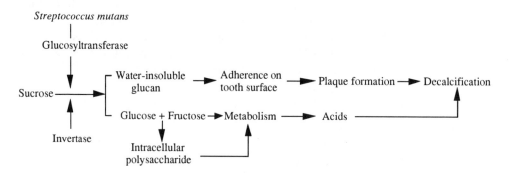

Figure 1. Proposed mechanism of dental caries formation.

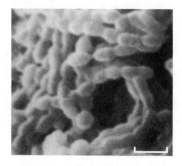

Figure 2. Scanning electron micrograph of *Streptococcus mutans*. Gram positive cocci, occuring in pairs, short or medium length chains. Bar = 1μm.

As mentioned above, the three major factors playing a key role in the occurrence of dental caries are host (tooth), bacteria, and substrate (sucrose) for the bacterial metabolism. Many studies carried out on these factors have been reported [10-13]. They are mainly about the strength of tooth surface, restriction or substitution of taking sucrose, and correlation between cariogenic bacterial cell contents and dental plaque.

The most traditional method of decreasing cariogenic bacteria and dental plaque is the mechanical control of using a dental brush or chemicals such as antibiotics, antibacterial substances, enzymes, or enzyme inhibitors, or their combination [14-16]. Various plant extracts have been investigated by many researchers aiming to prevent dental caries [17-19]. Comparing with the extracts so far examined, however, green tea polyphenols were found to be distinguishably effective for prevention of dental caries.

III. EFFECTS OF TEA POLYPHENOLS ON CARIOGENICITY OBSERVED IN *IN VITRO* TESTS

A. COMPONENTS OF TEA POLYPHENOLS AND THEIR EFFECTS ON GROWTH OF CARIOGENIC BACTERIA

1. Components of tea polyphenols

The tea polyphenols used here were those obtained by extracting dried green tea leaves with hot water, partitioning the water extract with ethyl acetate, and drying the solvent layer under reduced pressure.

The extract of green tea leaves inhibits the growth of cariogenic bacteria, *S. mutans* and *S. sobrinus*, and the degrees of the inhibition were in parallel with the concentration of the extract to be added. Also, the active principle was found to be tea polyphenols. The polyphenols were partitioned with several solvents into four fractions, and each active fraction was further partitioned on a silica gel column. Three peak fractions obtained were further fractionated by recycling on HPLC using a polyvinyl alcohol column (JAIGEL GS-320). Fraction 1 was separated into (+)-catechin (C) and (-)-epicatechin (EC) and fraction 2 into (+)-gallocatechin (GC), (-)-epigallocatechin (EGC), and (-)-epicatechin gallate (ECg) (Figure 3). Fraction 3 was identified to be (-)-epigallocatechin gallate (EGCg). Each isolated compound was identified based on the spectral evidences [6].

2. Inhibitory activities of polyphenol compounds

The minimum inhibitory concentrations (MICs) of each of the isolated tea polyphenols against cariogenic bacteria were determined as shown in Table 1. GC and EGC of concentrations between 250 and 500 μg/ml completely inhibited the growth of ten strains of cariogenic bacteria incubated on the brain heart infusion (BHI) medium. MIC of EGCg, which is a major component of tea polyphenols, was 1,000 μg/ml in the test on BHI. Their growth inhibitory effects were enhanced two-fold or more when examined using sensitive meat extract medium, and MIC of EGCg was 500 μg/ml. The inhibitory activities of GC and EGC were stronger than those of C and EC, and those of EGCg were the same as or slightly higher than ECg. These facts indicate that the presence of three hydroxyl groups at 3', 4', and 5' on the B ring in catechin and epicatechin molecules contribute to strengthen the inhibitory activity [6].

The MIC from 250-1000 μg/ml observed for tea polyphenols in the above-mentioned experiment is much higher in amount than various antibiotics. However, it is noteworthy that the green tea infusion for drinking usually contains 50-100 mg of the polyphenols per 100 ml [20] showng the richness of tea polyphenols in tea extract.

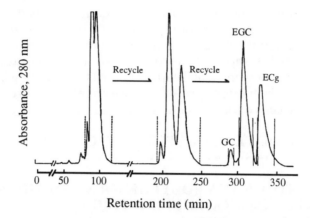

Figure 3. Isolation of components of green tea polyphenols by recycling HPLC. Column, JAIGEL GS-320 (50 cm × 2 cm); eluent, MeOH; flow rate, 3 ml/min; detector, UV at 280 nm; injection amount, 180 mg of fraction 2 eluted from a silica gel column. GC, EGC, and ECg were thus isolated. Reproduced from Sakanaka et al. (1989) [6] by permission of the Japan Society for Bioscience, Biotechnology, and Agrochemistry, Tokyo.

Table 1
MIC of Tea Polyphenols Isolated for Several Cariogenic Bacteria

Strains (serotype)		Test compound (μg/ml)					
		C	EC	GC	EGC	ECg	EGCg
E49	(a)	>1000	>1000	500	500	>1000	1000
		>1000	>1000	250	500	>1000	500
FA1	(b)	>1000	>1000	250	500	>1000	1000
		>1000	>1000	250	250	1000	500
MT8148	(c)	>1000	>1000	250	500	>1000	1000
		>1000	>1000	250	250	1000	500
IFO13955	(c)	>1000	>1000	250	500	>1000	1000
		>1000	>1000	250	250	>1000	500
MT4502	(d)	>1000	>1000	500	500	>1000	1000
		>1000	>1000	250	250	>1000	500
MT4245	(e)	>1000	>1000	250	500	>1000	1000
		>1000	>1000	250	250	1000	500
MT4251	(f)	>1000	>1000	250	500	>1000	1000
		>1000	>1000	250	250	1000	500
6715DP	(g)	>1000	>1000	250	500	>1000	1000
		>1000	>1000	250	250	>1000	500
MT4532	(g)	>1000	>1000	250	500	>1000	1000
		>1000	>1000	250	250	1000	500
MFe28	(h)	>1000	>1000	500	500	>1000	1000
		>1000	>1000	250	250	>1000	500

The upper and lower numbers are the results examined on BHI and sensitive meat extract agar medium, respecitvely.

B. INHIBITORY EFFECTS OF TEA POLYPHENOLS ON ENZYMIC SYNTHESIS OF GLUCANS AND ADHERENCE OF BACTERIAL CELLS ON TOOTH SURFACE

Cariogenic bacteria, *S. mutans* and *S. sobrinus*, synthesize water soluble and insoluble glucans by glucosyltransferase (GTase). GTases also synthesize an adherent, water-insoluble, and highly branched glucan which is responsible for the bacterial cell adherence to tooth surface [9].

Table 2 shows the effects of each component of green tea polyphenols on water-soluble and -insoluble glucan synthesis by the bacterial enzymes [7]. ECg, GCg, and EGCg strongly inhibit the glucan synthesis by any of the GTases examined. The degrees of inhibition of glucan synthesis by ECg and EGCg are almost proportional to their concentrations added, irrespective of the concentration of sucrose. As shown in Figure 4, both ECg and EGCg of concentrations more than 25-30 µg/ml almost completely inhibit glucan synthesis by the enzymes from *S. sobrinus* 6715DP and *S. mutans* MT8148 strains. Other polyphenols are not as inhibitory as ECg and EGCg.

The results of the effects of ECg and EGCg on adherence of *S. mutans* MT 8148 and *S. sobrinus* 6715DP are shown in Figure 5. The bacterial adherence onto glass surfaces has been reported to be due to the physical properties of glucans produced by the cell-bound GTases. Figure 5 indicates that both ECg and EGCg of concentrations of 50 µg/ml almost completely inhibit the adherence of the bacterial cells onto a glass surface [7].

Table 2

Inhibitory Effects of Tea Polyphenols on Glucosyltransferase Activity

Test compounds concentration µg/ml	Enzyme sources					
	6715DP		MT8148 GTase-I*		MT8148 GTase-S*	
	250	500	250	500	250	500
None	100	100	100	100	100	100
C	96.7**	73.1	83.7	61.2	95.0	71.0
EC	85.4	71.2	81.4	72.1	56.9	43.8
GC	31.7	9.7	97.2	85.8	82.7	61.8
EGC	84.7	61.0	94.0	82.0	96.4	58.7
ECg	≒0	≒0	≒0	≒0	≒0	≒0
GCg	≒0	≒0	≒0	≒0	≒0	≒0
EGCg	≒0	≒0	≒0	≒0	≒0	≒0

*GTase-I and GTase-S synthesize insoluble- and soluble-glucan, respectively.
**Values indicate relative activities of glucosyltransferase to the control determined without addition of the test compounds.
Reproduced from Sakanaka et al. (1990) [7] by permission of the Japan Society for Bioscience, Biotechnology, and Agrochemistry, Tokyo.

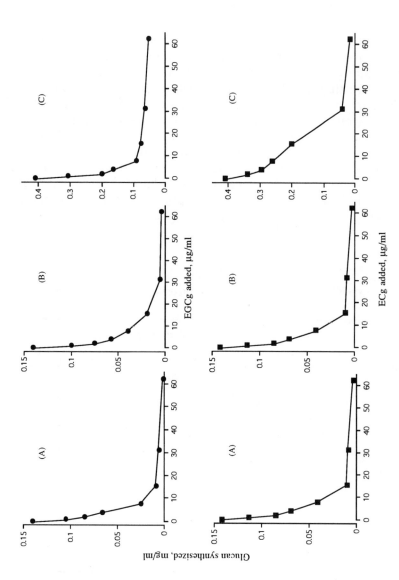

Figure 4. Effects of EGCg and ECg on enzymatic glucan synthesis. Sucrose concentration, 41.7 mM; (A) GTase from *S. sobrinus* 6715DP; (B) GTase-I from *S. mutans* MT8148; (C) GTase-S from *S. mutans* MT8148. ●, EGCg added; ■, ECg added. Reproduced from Sakanaka et al. (1990) [7] by permission of the Japan Society for Bioscience, Biotechnology, and Agrochemistry, Tokyo.

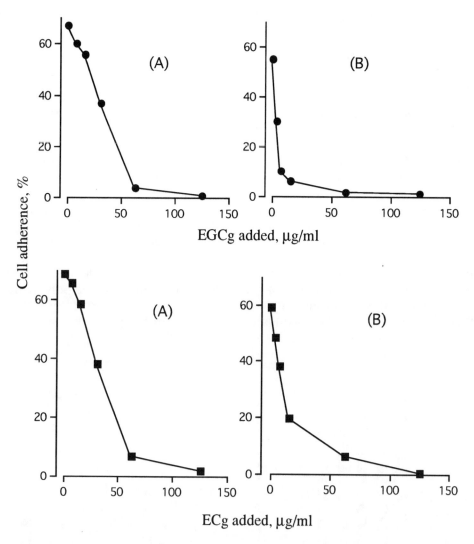

Figure 5. Effects of EGCg and ECg on adherence to glass surface of resting cells of S. mutans MT8148 and S. sobrinus 6715DP. Conditions: pH 6.8, 37°C, 18 hr; angle of incubation mixture, 30°; sucrose (20 mg) and S. sobrinus 6715DP (A) or S. mutans MT8148 (B) cells (1.0 mg as dry weight) in total 2.4 ml incubation mixture.
●, EGCg; ■, ECg. Reproduced from Sakanaka et al. (1990) [7] by permission of the Japan Society for Bioscience, Biotechnology, and Agrochemistry, Tokyo.

The concentrations of polyphenols effective to inhibit the enzymic synthesis of glucan or cellular adherence of the bacteria are less than those necessary to inhibit the bacterial growth. The most effective compounds are ECg and EGCg, both of which have galloyl moiety linked by ester linkage. Nevertheless, gallic acid itself is not inhibitory. Therefore, it is highly likely that the inhibitory effect shown by ECg and EGCg is attributed to their molecular configurations including the ester-linked galloyl moiety.

IV. EFFECTS OF TEA POLYPHENOLS ON DENTAL CARIES AND PLAQUES

A. EFFECTS ON DENTAL CARRIES IN RATS

Dental caries of both animals and humans are causally associated with the indigenous cariogenic streptococci in their mouths [21]. Sucrose is the main factor of food for bacterial virulence responsible for their cariogenicity. Sucrose is the substrate of the bacterial growth and synthesis of insoluble glucan by which the bacteria adhere to teeth surfaces. The green tea polyphenols were thus found to inhibit the bacterial growth, glucan synthesis, and cellular adherence of cariogenic streptococci *in vitro* test [6, 7].

The relationship between tea polyphenols administrated and dental caries in rats is as follows. The dental caries in rats were induced by the indigenous cariogenic bacteria on a sucrose diet. As shown in Figure 6, the addition of tea polyphenols to diet or to drinking water greatly reduced the inducement of caries. The addition of tea polyphenols to diet was more effective than that of the drinking water. It is likely that the constant cariogenic challenge presented by diet impacted into the sulti was overcome by the addition of tea polyphenols to the diet. Plates 8-10 following page 36 are a visual comparison of teeth of rats fed on cariogenic diets with and without (control) tea polyphenols [8].

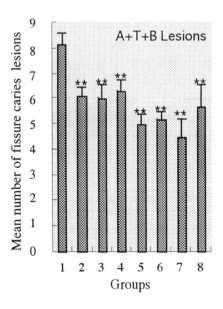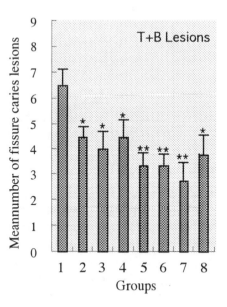

Figure 6. Mean number of fissure caries lesions in rats examined with or without tea polyphenols (TP). A, enamel lesions; T, lesions reaching the dentinoenamel junction; B, advanced dentin lesions. 1, control; 2, 0.1% TP in drinking water; 3, 0.2% TP in drinking water; 4, 0.5% TP in drinking water; 5, 0.1% TP in diet; 6, 0.2% TP in diet; 7, 0.5% TP in diet; 8, 0.1% TP in drinking water and 0.2% TP in diet. Data represent means ± SD.
*, $p < 0.05$; **, $p < 0.01$, compared with the control group using Student's t-test.
Reproduced from Sakanaka et al. (1992) [8] by permission of the Japan Society for Bioscience, Biotechnology, and Agrochemistry, Tokyo.

Table 3
Mandibular Mean Caries Scores of JCL-SD Rats Infected with S. mutans JC-2 (c) and Fed with Diet 2000 and Drinking Water with or without Tea Polyphenols (Sunphenon[R])

Group	Concentration of tea polyphenols in diet 2000, %	Concentration of tea polyphenols in drinking water, %	Mean (±SE) caries score [*]			
			sulcal	buccal	approximal	total
A	0	0	84.1±4.1	15.1±3.0	10.0±1.8	109.3±8.6
B	0.025	0	66.0±3.7**	18.7±2.7	9.3±1.3	94.0±7.3
C	0.05	0	55.1±3.7***	6.3±2.5***	3.1±1.2***	64.6±6.8**
D	0.1	0	54.7±3.9***	6.4±1.0***	3.1±0.7**	64.3±4.8**
E	0	0.025	67.7±2.9***	18.4±5.7	9.9±1.0	96.0±8.1
F	0	0.5	54.3±5.9**	8.9±3.7	3.0±1.3**	66.1±9.2**
G	0	0.1	55.4±3.6**	8.6±2.5	3.9±0.7***	67.9±6.1**
H	0.05	0.05	52.6±3.7**	10.6±2.8	3.7±0.9	66.9±7.0**

[*] Caries scores were determined in rats aged 78 days by the method of Keyes [23]. Statistical analysis (*t*-test) was carried out between group A and the other groups.
** p<0.01.
*** p<0.05.
Reproduced from Otake et al. (1991) [22] by permission of S. Karger AG, Basel.

Another experiment separately performed showed that when specific pathogen-free rats infected with *S. mutans* (sero type c) were given a diet or drinking water containing tea polyphenols of concentrations of more than 0.05%, the mean caries scores were significantly lower than those of the rats fed without tea polyphenols (Table 3). Thus, tea polyphenols were proved to be effective to reduce caries on sulcal, buccal, and approximal surfaces [22].

B. EFFECTS OF TEA POLYPHENOLS ON PLAQUE FORMATION IN MEN

The clinical efficacy of green tea polyphenols for prevention of dental plaque formation was investigated applying the cross-over, double-blind study [24]. The volunteers were 26 adult males of 23 to 35 years old (mean age, 26.5 years). The subjects who had received dental treatment or had any oral abnormalities at the time of this study were excluded.

After dental plaque in the subjects was completely removed using a dental pick, the subjects were made to rinse their mouths with 15 ml of water as a control solution or with a solution containing 0.05-0.5% of green tea polyphenols for 20 seconds. They performed the gargling three times a day immediately after meals during three consecutive days. The teeth after this three day treatment were taken as the control of individual subject. The subjects were forbidden to brush with any toothpaste or other tooth cleaner during the test period. After the control treatment, they were divided into four groups and made to rinse their mouths with 0.05, 0.1, 0.2, or 0.5% green tea polyphenols solutions, respectively, for the following three days. Immediately after this three days previous treatment, saliva and dental plaques of the subjects were collected, and the saliva samples were subjected to estimation of concentrations of lactic acid while the dental plaques for total bacterial cell counts were determined. The dental plaque was suspended in 5 ml sterile saline, and the total bacterial cells, streptococci, and lactobacilli, were determined by using BHI, MS, and LBS agar medium, respectively.

The dental plaque formation was identified by staining with Prospec dye. The stained upper and lower teeth were photographed, since the degree of dental plaque formation is known to correlate with the extent of color density developed by the staining. The photograph of each tooth was sectioned into four parts, and each part was evaluated based on the following criteria and compared with the control. The evaluation criteria were: 1) increase in the degree of staining, 2) no difference compared with control, and 3) decrease in the degree of staining.

The rate of inhibition against dental plaque formation was calculated by the following formula:

Inhibition rate (%) = (K-L)/M x 100, where
K, counts of the parts which decreased in the dental plaque formation;
L, counts of the parts which increased in the dental plaque formation;
M, counts of the total parts employed.

As shown in Table 4, the dental plaque formations decreased in the volunteers who rinsed with the solutions containing 0.05, 0.1, 0.2, or 0.5% green tea polyphenols. The inhibition rate of the dental plaque formation was

30-43% in the test groups. A visual comparison of the teeth of the subjects rinsed with and without (control) tea polyphenols is shown in Plates 8-10 following page 36.

The total cellular counts of bacteria and total streptococci in the dental plaque were also decreased in all the test groups. Significant differences were found in the 0.05% group ($p<0.01$) and 0.2% group ($p<0.05$). But, the total cellular counts of lactobacilli were almost the same between the two groups. The concentration of lactic acid in saliva decreased after rinsing with green tea polyphenols solutions in all the test groups.

It can be concluded from the above-mentioned results that green tea polyphenols act as an inhibitory agent for dental plaque formation and to decrease total bacteria and streptococci in a human mouth by rinsing with the solution.

Table 4
Effect of Tea Polyphenols on Dental Plaque Formation*

Groups	Concentration of tea polyphenols (%)	K	L	M	Inhibition rate (%)
I	0.05	53.5	12.5	100	41.0
II	0.1	43.2	9.3	100	33.9
III	0.2	38.6	8.0	100	30.6
IV	0.5	46.9	3.8	100	43.1
Mean		45.6	8.4	100	37.2

*See the text.
K, Counts of the parts which decreased in the dental plaque formation (%);
L, Counts of the parts which increased in the dental plaque formation (%);
M, Counts of the total parts employed (%).

C. EPIDEMIOLOGICAL SURVEY OF THE EFFECT OF GREEN TEA DRINKING FOR DENTAL CARIES RISK IN MEN

School children of the tea plantation area in Japan have been reported to be lower in the caries incidence as compared with those of other districts. The epidemiological studies were carried out using tea leaves containing a high content of fluoride and the effect of drinking the tea extract for caries prevention [25]. The investigation was carried out continuing over five years for the children of two primary schools which were selected from two typical Japanese farm villages. The average number of carious lesions in both schools decreased in the first program year, and the decreasing rates continued almost constantly. The decreasing rates in average were 22.1% in pit fissure and 26.1% in approximal sites. The results were those obtained when the children were made to drink only a cup of tea (Bancha) after school lunch and indicated that the tea infusion is an effective drink for prevention of dental caries. A similar result has been reported that tea drinking (1-3 cups/ day) resulted in a reduction of DMFT (the sum of decayed, missing, and filled teeth) and plaque score in school children of the U.S.A. [26]. The effect of green tea for prevention of dental caries was once thought to be due to fluorides contained in the tea leaves. However, the researchers noticed that the tea infusion was more effective for decreasing caries than a solution containing sodium fluoride alone [5]. This fact suggested that the tea infusion contains certain substances other than fluorides effective for prevention of dental caries.

V. RECENT TRENDS AND FUTURE ASPECTS OF THE APPLICATION OF GREEN TEA POLYPHENOLS

Recently, various sweetening agents have been developed as a substitute for sucrose [27, 28]. Nevertheless, sucrose has still been used because of the superior quality in the sweetness and thus, even now, it is much more popular than other sweeteners. Therefore, tea polyphenols have come to be applied for confectioneries using sucrose such as chewing gums, candies, caramels, jelly beans, beverages, and several other products in Japan, as a dental carries prevention agent. The application of tea polyphenols have been based on the following findings. Chocolates, candies, caramels, biscuits, etc. sweetened with sucrose and with or without tea polyphenols were prepared and fed to rats to examine the incidence of dental caries. The rats used were previously infected with *S. mutans*. The result showed that the dental caries score was distinctly lower in rats fed with the confectionaries with tea polyphenols (Figure 7) [29]. It has also been reported that chewing gum added with tea polyphenols is effective in decreasing dental plaque formation in humans [30].

The complete prevention of dental caries has not been established yet, because dental caries formation involves many interrelated factors. In recent years, much attention has been focused on green tea for its various medical effects. Polyphenolic compounds are found to exist in various plants, and some of them may also possess the potential anticariogenic activities such as growth inhibition and depression of glucan synthesis [17-19]. Several papers published so far have also reported tea polyphenols to be significantly effective in inhibition of dental and enamel caries [31].

Green tea polyphenols are characteristic in a remarkably strong inhibition activity of glucan synthesis. The strongest inhibitory activity was observed with ECg, EGCg, and GCg. Similar results have been reported on gallotannins isolated from *Melaphis chinensis* which inhibits GTase activity of *S. sobrinus* [32]. These facts clearly indicate that the polyphenolic compounds having galloyl groups exhibit a strong GTase inhibition activity.

The test of rinsing the mouth with the water containing green tea polyphenols also resulted in significant reduction in dental plaque formation in men. It should be noted that the concentration of tea polyphenols in green tea infusion is quite effective since 100 ml of green tea infusion contains approximately 50-100 mg of tea polyphenols [20]. Also, it was mentioned that a cup of green tea after lunch resulted in a reduction of dental caries risk in school children [25]. As described in other chapters of this book, green tea polyphenols are quite safe as food additives. Furthermore, green tea polyphenols were clarified to exhibit several other physiological and biochemical activities as well as prevention of dental carries. Therefore, the application of green tea polyphenols seems to have great potential to be further developed as an additive to various foods.

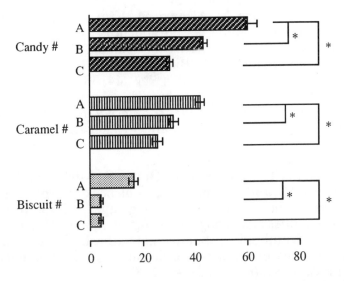

Figure 7. Total of mean caries scores of SPF rats infected with *S. mutans* JC-2 (c) and fed with diet M2000.
#: 56% sucrose in diet 2000 was replaced with candy, caramel, or biscuit, and the sucrose concentration of each preparation was 31%, 14%, and 9%, respectively.
A, Control; B, containing 0.1% tea polyphenols (Sunphenon^R); C, containing 0.2% tea polyphenols (Sunphenon^R).
*Significance of difference, $p < 0.01$.
Reproduced from Nishihara et al. (1993) [29] by permission of Nihon University, Tokyo.

REFERENCES

1. **Sanderson, G. W.,** The chemistry of tea and tea manufacturing, *Rec. Adv. Phytochemistry*, **5**, 247, 1972.
2. **Bokuchava, M. A. and Skobeleva, N. I.,** The biochemistry and technology of tea manufacture, *CRC Critical Reviews in Food Science and Nutriton*, **12**, 303, 1980.
3. **Onisi, M., Okumura, F., and Murakami, Y.,** *In vitro* screening of tea leaves effective against dental caries, *J. Dent. Hlth.*, **27**, 279, 1978.
4. **Onisi, M., Shimura, N., Nakamura, C., and Sato, M.,** A field test on the caries preventive effect of tea drinking, *J. Dent. Hlth.*, **31**, 13, 1981.
5. **Onisi, M., Ozaki, F., Yoshino, F., and Murakami, Y.,** An experimental evidence of caries preventive activity of non-fluoride component in tea, *J. Dent. Hlth.*, **31**, 158, 1981.

6. **Sakanaka, S., Kim, M., Taniguchi, M., and Yamamoto, T.,** Antibacterial substances in Japanese green tea extract against *Streptococcus mutans*, a cariogenic bacterium, *Agric. Biol. Chem.*, **53**, 2307, 1989.
7. **Sakanaka, S., Sato, T., Kim, M., and Yamamaoto, T.,** Effects of green tea polyphenols on glucan synthesis and cellular adherence of cariogenic streptococci, *Agric. Biol. Chem.*, **54**, 2925, 1990.
8. **Sakanaka, S., Shimura, N., Aizawa, M., Kim, M., and Yamamoto, T.,** Preventive effect of green tea polyphenols against dental caries in conventional rats, *Biosci. Biotech. Biochem.*, **56**, 592, 1992.
9. **Hamada, S. and Slade, H. D.,** Biology, immunology, and cariogenicity of *Streptococcus mutans*, *Microbiol. Rev.*, **44**, 331, 1980.
10. **Takeuchi, M.,** Epidemiological study on dental caries in Japanese children before, during and after World War II, *Internat. Dent. J.*, **11**, 443, 1961.
11. **Littleton, N. W., Kakehashi, S., and Fitzgerald, R. J.,** Recovery of specific "caries-inducing" streptococci from caries lesions in the teeth of child, *Arch. Oral Biol.*, **15**, 461, 1970.
12. **Ikeda, T., Shiota, T., Mcghee, J. R., Otake, S., Michalek, S. M., Ochiai, K., Hirasawa, M., and Sugimoto, K.,** Virulence of *Streptococcus mutans*. Comparison of the effects of a coupling sugar and sucrose on certain metabolic activities and cariogenicity, *Infect. Immun.*, **19**, 477, 1978.
13. **Ooshima, T., Izumitani, A., Sobue, S., Okahashi, N., and Hamada, S.,** Non-cariogenicity of the disaccharide palatinose in experimental dental caries of rats, *Infect. Immun.*, **39**, 43, 1983.
14. **Baker, P. J., Slots, J., Genco, R. J., and Evans, R. T.,** Minimal inhibitory concentrations of various antimicrobial agents for human oral anaerobic bacteria, *Antimicrob. Agents Chemother.*, **24**, 420, 1983.
15. **Saeki, Y., Ito, Y., Shibata, M., Sato, Y., Okuda, K., and Takazoe, I.,** Antibacterial action of natural substances on oral bacteria, *Bull. Tokyo Dent. Coll.*, **30**, 129, 1989.
16. **Okami, Y., Takashio, M., and Umezawa, H.,** Ribocitorin, a new inhibitor of dextransucrase, *J. Antibiot.*, **24**, 344, 1981.
17. **Kakiuchi, N., Hattori, M., Nishizawa, M., Yamagishi, T., Okuda, T., and Namba, T.,** Studies on dental caries prevention by traditional medicines. VIII. Inhibitory effect of various tannins on glucan synthesis by glucosyltransferase from *Streptococcus mutans*, *Chem. Pharm. Bull.*, **34**, 720, 1986.
18. **Heisey, R. M. and Gorham, B. K.,** Antimicrobial effects of plant extracts on *Streptococcus mutans*, *Candida albicans*, *Tricophyton rubrum* and other microorganisms, *Lett. Appl. Microbiol.*, **14**, 136, 1992.
19. **Wolinsky, L. E. and Sote, E. O.,** Isolation of natural plaque-inhibiting substances from 'Nigerian chewing sticks', *Caries Res.*, **18**, 216, 1984.
20. **Maeda, S. and Nakagawa, M.,** General chemical and physical analysis on various kinds of green tea, *Chagyo Kenkyu Hokoku (in Japanese)*, **45**, 85, 1977.
21. **Loesche, W. J.,** Role of *Streptococcus mutans* in human dental decay, *Microbiol. Rev.*, **50**, 353, 1986.
22. **Otake, S., Makimura, M., Kuroki, T., Nishihara, Y., and Hirasawa, M.,** Anticaries effects of polyphenolic compounds from Japanese green tea, *Caries Res.*, **25**, 438, 1991.

23. **Keyes, P. H.**, Dental caries in the molar teeth of rats, *J. Dent. Res.*, **37**, 1088, 1958.
24. **Oiwa, T., Sakanaka, S., Kim, M., Ozaki, T., Kashiwagi, M., Hasegawa, Y., Yoshihara, Y., and Yoshida, S.**, Inhibitory effect of human plaque formation by green tea polyphenols (Sunphenon), *Jpn. J. Prd. Dent. (in Japanese)*, **31**, 247, 1993.
25. **Onisi, M.**, The feasibility of a tea drinking program for dental public health in primary schools, *J. Dent. Hlth.*, **35**, 402, 1985.
26. **Elvin-Lewis, M. and Steelman, R.**, The anticariogenic effects of tea drinking among Dallas school children, *J. Dent. Res.*, **65**, 198, 1986.
27. **Edgar, W. M. and Dodds, M. W. J.**, The effect of sweetners on acid production in plaque, *Int. Dent. J.*, **35**, 18, 1985.
28. **Imfeld, T. N.**, Clinical caries studies with polyalcohols, *Schweiz Monatsschr Zahnmed*, **104**, 941, 1994.
29. **Nishihara, Y., Aori, T., Ohkawa, T., Wada, Y., Makimura, M., Hirasawa, M., and Otake, S.**, Inhibitory effects of food containing sucrose added tea catechins on dental caries in rats, *Nihon Univ. J. Oral Sci. (in Japanese)*, **19**, 217, 1993.
30. **Sakanaka, S., Mamiya, S., Kim, M., Itoh, K., Otomo, Y., and Miyaaki, T.**, Inhibitory effect of tea polyphenols and lactitol on human dental plaque formation, *Abstracts of Papers, Annual Meeting of Agric. Chem. Soc. of Japan*, 1996, p 9.
31. **Rosen, S., Elvin-Lewis, M., Beck, F. M., and Beck, E. X.**, Anticariogenic effects of tea in rats, *J. Dent. Res.*, **63**, 658, 1984.
32. **Wu-Yuan, C. D., Chen, C. Y., and Wu, R. T.**, Gallotannins inhibit growth, water-insoluble glucan synthesis, and aggregation of mutans streptococci, *J. Dent. Res.*, **67**, 51, 1988.

Chapter 9

INHIBITORY EFFECTS OF GREEN TEA POLYPHENOLS ON GROWTH AND CELLULAR ADHERENCE OF PERIODONTAL DISEASE BACTERIUM, *PORPHYROMONAS GINGIVALIS*

S. Sakanaka and T. Yamamoto

TABLE OF CONTENTS

I. Introduction
II. Inhibitory Effect of Tea Polyphenols on Growth of *P. gingivalis*
    A. Inhibitory Effect on Adherence of *P. gingivalis* onto Buccal Epithelial Cells
    B. Effect of Components of Tea Polyphenols on Adherence of *P. gingivalis* onto Buccal Epithelial Cells
III. Influence of EGCg on Adherence of Other Bacterial Cells onto Oral Epithelial Cells
References

I. INTRODUCTION

Periodontal disease brings an inflammatory and destructive lesion in the periodontal tissue. This disease is known to be caused by subgingival plaque bacteria. *Porphyromonas gingivalis* has been isolated as the bacterium most frequently found in the subgingival plaque of patients with advanced adult periodontitis [1, 2]. *P. gingivalis* adheres onto our oral epithelial cells [3]. Adherence of bacteria onto their host tissue cells is the first step of bacterial infection. The adhered bacteria begin their growth, colonization, and production of virulent factors which injure the host tissue cells [4]. The property of *P. gingivalis* to adhere onto oral epithelial cells may be correlated with the virulent factors of periodontal pathogens.

It has been reported that monoclonal antibodies against the fimbriae of *P. gingivalis* specifically inhibit the adherence of *P. gingivalis* onto the epithelial cells [5]. However, no paper has been published on demonstration of the inhibitory effect of components found in foods on adherence of *P. gingivalis* onto epithelial cells.

Our recent studies on the relationship between Japanese green tea and dental caries, showed that green tea polyphenols decreased the caries risk in the experiments by both the *in vitro* and *in vivo* tests [6-8]. We also reported that green tea polyphenols (tea catechins) inhibit the activity of collagenase known as one of the virulent factors of periodontal disease [9]. In this chapter, the effect of green tea polyphenols on adherence of *P. gingivalis* onto human buccal epithelial cells is described, showing the evidence that green tea polyphenols, especially (-)-epigallocatechin gallate, (-)-gallocatechin gallate, and (-)-epicatechin gallate, strongly inhibit the adherence of the bacterium [10].

Recently, Katoh (1995) reported that in the experiment using mice infected with *Actinomyces viscosus* the occurrence of periodontal disease was greatly reduced by administration of tea polyphenols through diet or drinking water [11].

II. INHIBITORY EFFECT OF TEA POLYPHENOLS ON GROWTH OF *P. GINGIVALIS*

The effects of each component of tea polyphenols on the growth of several strains of *Porphyromonas* are shown in Table 1. Among several tea polyphenols examined, EGCg which is the dominant component of green tea polyphenols, completely inhibited the growth of three strains of *P. gingivalis* at concentrations of 250 or 500 µg/ml, though the effective concentrations are much larger as compared with various antibiotics known so far. EGCg also inhibited the growth of *P. melaninogenicus*, but its minimum inhibitory concentration (MIC) was 2000 µg/ml.

Table 1

Minimum Inhibitory Concentrations of Tea Polyphenols for the Growth of Several Oral Bacteria*

Strains	Test compounds					
	C(+)	EC	GC	EGC	ECg	EGCg
Porphyromonas gingivalis 381	1000**	1000	1000	1000	1000	500
Porphyromonas gingivalis ATCC 33277	1000	1000	1000	1000	1000	250
Porphyromonas gingivalis GAI 7802	1000	1000	1000	1000	1000	500
Porphyromonas melaninogenicus GAI 5596	>2000	>2000	>2000	>2000	>2000	2000

*The bacteria were anaerobically grown on general anaerobic medium containing 1.5% agar and varied concentrations of compounds at 37°C for 48 hr, and their growth was visually compared.

** µg/ml

Reproduced from Sakanaka et al. (1996) [10] by permission of the Japan Society for Bioscience, Biotechnology, and Agrochemistry, Tokyo.

A. INHIBITORY EFFECT ON ADHERENCE OF *P. GINGIVALIS* ONTO BUCCAL EPITHELIAL CELLS

P. gingivalis isolated from human subgingival plaque is a typical bacterium that adheres onto our oral epithelial cells. As can be seen from Figure 1, the cells of *P. gingivalis* usually observed per an oral epithelial cell of healthy males are about 200 in average. However, the presence of tea polyphenols decreased the number adhered to cells in a dose-dependent manner. At the concentration of 50 µg/ml of tea polyphenols, the adherence of bacterial cells onto buccal epithelial cells was inhibited almost completely.

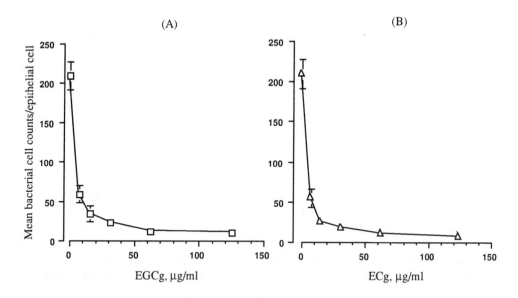

Figure 1. Inhibitory effect of EGCg and ECg on adherence of *P. gingivalis* 381 onto human buccal epithelial cells. *P. gingivalis* 381 and epithelial cells were incubated at 37°C for 60 min with EGCg or ECg at various concentrations and washed five times by centrifugation (1000 rpm, 3 min) with 0.1 M Na-phosphate buffer (pH 6.0). The epithelial cells were then smeared on a glass slide, dried, and stained with a safranin solution. The bacterial cells adhered onto 20 epithelial cells were counted by light microscopy. Each value represents the mean ±standard error. Reproduced from Sakanaka et al. (1996) [10] by permission of the Japan Society for Bioscience, Biotechnology, and Agrochemistry, Tokyo.

B. EFFECT OF COMPONENTS OF TEA POLYPHENOLS ON ADHERENCE OF *P. GINGIVALIS* ONTO BUCCAL EPITHELIAL CELLS

As shown in Figure 2, all the components of green tea polyphenols and ethyl gallate (Eg) employed as a reference (250 µg/ml) inhibited adherence of *P. gingivalis* onto epithelial cells. However, EGCg, GCg, and ECg, all of which have galloyl moiety linked by ester linkage, were pronounced in the inhibitory effect. At the concentration of 250 µg/ml, they inhibited the adherence of *P. gingivalis* almost completely. On the other hand, C, EC, GC, EGC, and Eg were not so effective as galloyl polyphenols at the same concentrations.

The inhibitory effect of galloyl polyphenols on the bacterial adherence was thought to be attributed to the sensitivity of the bacterium to those compounds, because the degree of adherence of *P. gingivalis* onto the epithelial cells which were previously incubated with EGCg for 15 min was about 70% of the control run; whereas the adherence of the bacterial cells previously incubated with EGCg for 15 min was greatly affected, and the degree of the adherence was only about 25% of the control.

III. INFLUENCE OF EGCg ON ADHERENCE OF OTHER BACTERIAL CELLS ONTO ORAL EPITHELIAL CELLS

The adherence of EGCg onto the oral epithelial cells has been observed so far with several bacteria. In our experiment, *Porphyromonas* species were distinguished in the adherence onto epithelial cells with considerably high ratios. Other bacteria were less than 200 cells per epithelial cell. It should be noted that the bacteria, such as *Clostridium*, *Escherichia*, and *Bacillus* species, are usually not found in our oral cavity.

Table 2 shows that the inhibitory effect of EGCg on the adherence of various bacteria onto epithelial cells. The addition of EGCg at 125 µg/ml resulted in almost complete inhibition of adherence of *Porphyromonas* species. However, unlike the case of *P. gingivalis*, the adherence of other bacteria, such as *Streptococcus salivalius*, *Streptococcus sanguis*, and *Staphylococcus aureus*, was not so drastically inhibited by EGCg. This finding is an interesting and important indication that the mechanism involved in adherence onto epithelial cells is different at least between *P. gingivalis* and Streptococci or Staphylococci. The mechanism involved in adherence of *P. gingivalis* on buccal epithelial cells is under investigation and will be elucidated in the near future.

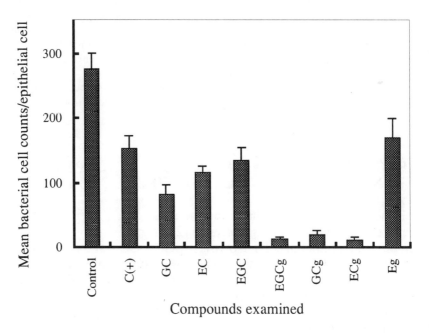

Figure 2. Inhibitory effect of tea polyphenols and ethyl gallate on adherence *P. gingivalis* 381 onto human buccal epithelial cells. *P. gingivalis* 381 and epithelial cells were incubated with the test compound (250 µg/ml). The adherence assay was carried out as described in Figure 1. Reproduced from Sakanaka et al. (1996) [10] by permission of the Japan Society for Bioscience, Biotechnology, and Agrochemistry, Tokyo.

Table 2
Diversity in Adherence of Various Bacteria onto Human Buccal Epithelial Cells and Inhibitory Effect of EGCg on Their Adherence Activity

Bacteria	EGCg (µg/ml)		
	0	125	250
Porphyromonas gingivalis 381	281.1± 25.8*	14.3± 3.1	11.7± 1.8
Porphyromonas gingivalis ATCC 33277	301.4± 51.9	19.5± 4.2	9.6± 2.0
Porphyromonas gingivalis GAI 7802	46.3± 7.2	2.7± 1.1	0.8± 0.5
Porphyromonas melaninogenicus GAI 5596	221.0± 27.7	16.4± 4.7	13.5± 4.2
Streptococcus mutans MT8148R	44.5± 6.8	16.9± 4.6	12.6± 6.0
Streptococcus salivalius JCM 5707	53.9± 10.5	34.0± 6.2	20.0± 3.3
Streptococcus sanguis JCM 5708	110.6± 24.2	65.4± 11.5	39.2± 5.8
Clostridium perfringens JCM 1290	2.9± 0.9	nd**	nd
Clostridium perfringens JCM 3817	0.5± 0.3	nd	nd
Escherichia coli IFO 3545	3.3± 1.2	1.7± 1.1	1.3± 0.4
Staphylococcus aureus IFO 12732	85.9± 14.5	60.2±12.4	41.2± 4.9
Bacillus subtilis IFO 3007	01.±0.1	nd	nd

*Each value represents the mean of bacterial cells adhered ± standard error per epithelial cell.
**Not done

Reproduced from Sakanaka et al. (1996) [10] by permission of the Japan Society for Bioscience, Biotechnology, and Agrochemistry, Tokyo.

REFERENCES

1. **Slot, J.,** The predominant cultivable microflora of advanced periodontitis, *J. Dent. Res.*, **85**, 114, 1977.
2. **Tanner, A. C. R., Haffer, C., Bratthall, G. T. R., Visconti, A., and Socransky, S. S.,** A study of the bacteria associated with advancing periodontitis in man, *J. Clin. Periodont.*, **6**, 278, 1979.
3. **Slot, J. and Gibbons, R. J.,** Attachment of *Bacteroides melaninogenicus* subsp. *asaccharolyticus* to oral surfaces and its possible role in colonization of the mouth and of periodontal pockets, *Infect. Immun.*, **19**, 254, 1978.
4. **Ofek, I. and Beachey, E. H.,** General concepts and principals of bacterial adherence in animals and man, in *Bacterial Adherence. Series B*, **Vol. 6**, Beachey, E. H., Ed., Chapman and Hall, London, 1980, p 1.
5. **Isogai, H., Isogai, E., Yoshimura, F., Suzuki, T., Kagota, W., and Takano, K.,** Specific inhibition of adherence of an oral strain of *Bacteroides gingivalis* 381 to epithelial cells by monoclonal antibodies against the bacterial fimbriae, *Archs. Oral Biol.*, **33**, 479, 1988.

6. **Sakanaka, S., Kim, M., Taniguchi, M., and Yamamoto, T.,** Antibacterial substances in Japanese green tea extract against *Streptococcus mutans*, a cariogenic bacterium, *Agric. Biol. Chem.*, **53**, 2307, 1989.
7. **Sakanaka, S., Sato, T., Kim, M., and Yamamoto, T.,** Inhibitory effects of green tea polyphenols on glucan synthesis and cellular adherence of cariogenic streptococci, *Agric. Biol. Chem.*, **54**, 2925, 1990.
8. **Sakanaka, S., Shimura, N., Aizawa, M., Kim, M., and Yamamoto, T.,** Preventive effect of green tea polyphenols against dental caries in conventional rats, *Biosci. Biotech. Biochem.*, **56**, 592, 1992.
9. **Makimura, M., Hirasawa, M., Kobayashi, K., Indo, J., Sakanaka, S., Taguchi, T., and Otake, S.,** Inhibitory effect of tea catechins on collagenase activity, *J. Periodontol.*, **64**, 630, 1993.
10. **Sakanaka, S., Aizawa, M., Kim, M., and Yamamoto, T.,** Inhibitory effects of green tea polyphenols on growth and cellular adherence of an oral bacterium, *Porphyromonas gingivalis*, *Biosci. Biotech. Biochem.*, **60**, 745, 1996.
11. **Katoh, H.,** Prevention of mouse experimental periodontal disease by tea catechins, *Nihon Univ. J. Oral Sci. (in Japanese)*, **21**, 1, 1995.

Chapter 10

EFFECTS OF GREEN TEA POLYPHENOLS ON HUMAN INTESTINAL MICROFLORA

T. Okubo and L. R. Juneja

TABLE OF CONTENTS

I. Introduction
II. Effect of Tea Polyphenols on Various Intestinal Microflora
III. Effects of Tea Polyphenols on Intestinal Microflora and Their Metabolites in Volunteers
IV. Antiviral Effect of Tea Polyphenols
References

I. INTRODUCTION

In our intestine, more than one hundred kinds of bacteria exist and their cellular counts amount to about a hundred trillion in total. These bacteria constitute a certain complicated flora ecologically. The foods we intake are enzymatically digested, and most of the digested products are absorbed during the passage from mouth to small intestine.

The undigested or unabsorbed substances, on the other hand, reach the large intestine where they are subjected to the action of various bacteria to produce their metabolites. These bacteria and their metabolites are known to be closely associated with our nutrition, health, aging, and certain diseases. For example, the acid forming bacteria such as certain *Bifidobacterium* and *Lactobacillus* genera bacteria are known to be useful to our health, because they synthesize several vitamins and act to stimulate digestion and absorption of the digestion products as nutrients or inhibit the growth of unfavorable germs [1, 2]. On the other hand, certain clostridia such as *Clostridium perfringens, C. difficile*, etc. have been inferred to be closely related with disturbance of intestinal condition, leading to the acceleration of aging or evolution of a tumor [3-5]. The microflora in our large intestine are always affected by external environmental factors. The composition of our diet is the most important factor affecting the microflora.

A number of papers have been published on the relationships between diet composition and intestinal microflora [6-8]. Formerly, our research group investigated the effects on intestinal microflora of ginseng extract [9], extract of several herbs or fruits with liquor, green tea extracts [10, 11], soluble plant heteropolysaccharides as fiber, etc. and reported that the extracts of *Panax ginseng* (*Araliaceae* family) enhance the growth of bifidobacteria while it selectively inhibits the growth of clostridia. Unlike an *in vitro* test, an *in vivo* test involves various factors which may influence each other. Therefore, the results obtained with an *in vivo* test must be analyzed carefully from various points for a conclusion.

This chapter describes the effects of green tea extract on microflora in our intestine, showing that the green tea extract brings several merits to our health through ecologically adjusting the intestinal microflora.

II. EFFECT OF TEA POLYPHENOLS ON VARIOUS INTESTINAL MICROFLORA

The hot water infusion of green tea leaves (*Camellia sinensis* L, *Theaceae* family) has long been loved as a habitual drink by the people of East Asia. The infusion is rich in several biologically active compounds such as caffeine, polyphenols, theanine, vitamins, saponins, etc. Many papers have reported that the green tea extract has antimutagenic [12, 13], hypolipemic [14], antitumor [15-18], antioxidative [19], and antibacterial activities [20, 21]. However, studies of the effects of green tea extract on the ecology of intestinal microflora and their metabolisms have remained undone so far. We studied the effects of green tea extract on the growth-response of various intestinal microorganisms [10].

As shown in Table 1, the addition of 0.1% of the methanol extract of green tea leaves, which was used after drying and pulverizing, to a modified Gyorgy broth as the culture medium induced a slight or moderate growth of *Bifidobacterium adolescentis* (strain E194a), *B. longum, B. breve, B. infantis, Lactobacillus casei,* and *L. salivarius*. But, it was not effective when used at concentrations of 1% (w/v) or more in the modified Gyorgy broth under which condition, the growth-response is to be due to several nutrients other than 0.5% glucose. Other bacteria, including clostridia and *E. coli*, were unable to grow in the presence of green tea extract. On the other hand, a moderate growth of three species of lactobacilli was shown when examined using 1% concentration of the tea extract in Peptone Yeast Fildes (PYF) broth.

Kakuda and his colleagues reported that the growth of *Bifidobacterium adolescentis* was enhanced by the presence of water extracts of green tea marketed as "Gyokuro" and "Sencha" with the concentration dependence, but *Clostridium perfringens, Bacteroides fragilis,* and *Eubacterium lentum* showed no growth promotion under the same conditions [22]. The crude extracts of Gyokuro were more effective in enhancing growth of bifidobacteria than Sencha at an equivalent concentration. They suggested that the enhancing effect of tea extract on the growth of bifidobacteria was a result due to the nutritive effects of the inorganic (potassium and phosphorus) and organic substances (several free amino acids and saccharides) contained in the extract.

The above-mentioned study supports our observation that the green tea extract promotes the growth of certain bifido- and lactic acid-forming bacteria, and the effective components seemed to us initially to be the same components as those suggested by Kakuda and his colleagues. However, in the study of the effects of green tea extract on various intestinal bacteria by the impregnated paper-disc method (10 mg tea extract/disc, 8 mm¢) [11], we found that the propagation of all clostridial species examined were inhibited with the exception of *Clostridium butyricum, C. coccoides,* and one of two strains of *C. ramosum* (strain C-00). The green tea extract, on the other hand, showed no growth inhibition against other bacteria examined in the same test method.

The green tea polyphenols which show a selective inhibition against clostridia consisted of the following six components: (+)-catechin, (-)-epicatechin, (+)-gallocatechin, (-)-epigallocatechin, (-)-epicatechin gallate, and (-)-epigallocatechin gallate. Table 2 shows the growth-inhibitory effects of the six polyphenols above against two strains of clostridia. The bacterial

Table 1
Growth Response and Inhibition by Green Tea Extract of Intestinal Microorganisms

Strain	Response		Inhibition
	PYF med.	Gyorgy med.	
Bifidobacterium adolescentis E-194a	-	+	-
B. adolescentis E-319a	-	+	-
B. bifidum E-319a	-	-	-
B. bifidum S-28a	-	-	-
B. breve S-1	-	+	-
B. breve S-46	-	+	-
B. infantis S-12	-	+	-
B. infantis 1-10-5	-	+	-
B. longum E-194b	-	+	-
B. longum Kd-5-6	-	+	-
Lactobacillus acidophilus ATCC-4356	+	-	-
L. casei ATCC-7469	+	+	-
L. salivarius ATCC-11741	+	+	-
Bacteroides distasonis B-26	-	-	-
B. distasonis S-601	-	-	-
B. fragilis M-601	-	-	-
B. fragilis VI-23	-	-	-
B. thetaiotaomicron AS-126	-	-	-
B. vulgatus B-24	-	-	-
B. vulgatus F-62	-	-	-
Clostridium bifermentans B-1	-	-	+
C. bifermentans B-4	-	-	+
C. butyricum ATCC-14823	-	-	-
C. butyricum S-601	-	-	-
C. coccoides B-2	-	-	-
C. difficile ATCC-9689	-	-	+
C. innocuum M-601	-	-	+
C. paraputrificum B-3-4	-	-	+
C. paraputrificum B-78	-	-	+
C. paraputrificum VPI-6372	-	-	+
C. perfringens ATCC-13124	-	-	+
C. perfringens B-3-7	-	-	+
C. perfringens B-3-8	-	-	+
C. perfringens B-165-16	-	-	+
C. perfringens C-01	-	-	+
C. ramosum ATCC-25582	-	-	+
C. ramosum C-00	-	-	-
Eubacterium aerofaciens S-601	-	-	-
E. aerofaciens S-605	-	-	-
E. lentum M-601	-	-	-
E. limosum E-1	-	-	-
Escherichia coli E-605	-	-	-
E. coli M-602	-	-	-
E. coli O-601	-	-	-
E. coli V-603	-	-	-

The test strains obtained from the RIKEN culture collection were cultured in PYF medium without supply of any carbon sources. The Gyorgy medium was supplied 0.5% glucose and 1% methanol extracts of green tea. Growth responses were scored as +, pH 5.1-5.5; -, no response. The inhibitory effects of green tea extract were assayed by the paper disc method using a paper disc (ϕ 8mm, Toyo Roshi, Japan) containing 10 mg green tea extract/disc on Brucella agar (Difco). All the tests of inhibition were done three times, and a mean inhibition zone of 12 mm or larger was estimated as +.

growth inhibition test was carried out by the paper disc method mentioned above. In the test using 5 mg/disc, (-)-epicatechin gallate and (-)-epigallocatechin gallate were strongest in growth inhibition while other polyphenols showed no inhibitory effects for the two clostridia. In the test against *C. perfringens*, (-)-epicatechin gallate and (-)-epigallocatechin gallate showed a strong growth inhibition. (+)-Catechin, (-)-epicatechin, and (+)-gallocatechin showed inhibition for the bacterium but not as strong as the two catechins above. (-)-Epigallocatechin showed no effect. These results suggest a certain relationship between the structures of polyphenols and the bacterial growth inhibitory effects. The gallate moiety linked by ester linkage in the polyphenol molecules seem to be related to the bacterial growth inhibition activity regardless of their stereotypes.

Table 2

Growth Inhibitory Activity of Tea Polyphenols
Against *C. difficile* ATCC-9689 and *C. perfringens* ATCC-13124

Test compound*	C. difficile			C. perfringens		
	0.5	1.0	5.0 mg/disc	0.5	1.0	5.0 mg/disc
C	-	-	-	-	-	+
EC	-	-	-	-	-	+
GC	-	-	-	-	-	+
ECg	-	-	++	-	-	++
EGC	-	-	-	-	-	-
EGCg	-	-	++	-	-	++

*Abbr.: C, (+)-catechin; EC, (-)-epicatechin; GC, (+)-gallocatechin; ECg, (-)-epicatechin gallate; EGC, (-)-epigallocataechin; EGCg, (-)-epigallocatechin gallate. Reproduced from Ahn et al. (1991) [11] by permission of the Japan Society for Bioscience, Biotechnology, and Agrochemistry, Tokyo.

III. EFFECTS OF TEA POLYPHENOLS ON INTESTINAL MICROFLORA AND THEIR METABOLITES IN VOLUNTEERS

As mentioned above, an *in vitro* test study showed that the methanol extract of green tea leaves enhanced the growth of some lactic acid forming bacteria, though the tea extract specifically inhibited several clostridial bacilli. The most inhibitory active compounds were the catechin derivatives having an ester-linked gallate moiety, and they showed a strong growth inhibition against *C. difficile* and *C. perfringens* as mentioned above.

Effects of tea polyphenols intake (0.4 g polyphenols of one dose, 3 times a day for 4 weeks total of 8 weeks) on fecal bacterial ecology, their metabolites, and pH of the feces were investigated for eight healthy volunteers [23]. The test was scheduled dividing the term into four consecutive periods. Control period A (1st and 2nd weeks, no administration), Test period 1 (3rd and 4th weeks, administrated), Test period 2 (5th and 6th weeks, administrated), and Control period B (7th and 8th weeks, no administration). Table 3 shows the effect of tea polyphenols intake on various intestinal microflora with their cellular counts.

Table 3
Effects of Tea Polyphenols on Intestinal Bacterial Cell Counts in Volunteers [1,2]

Microflora	Control A	Test 1	Test 2	Control B
Total	11.03±0.04	10.91±0.06	10.92±0.05	11.03±0.07
Bacteroidaceae	10.66±0.04	10.58±0.07	10.57±0.07	10.71±0.08
	(16/16)	(16/16)	(16/16)	(16/16)
Eubacterium spp.	10.44±0.06	10.38±0.06	10.39±0.05	10.43±0.31
	(16/16)	(16/16)	(16/16)	(16/16)
Peptococcaeceae	9.88±0.10	9.59±0.16	9.43±0.15	9.62±0.13
	(16/16)	(15/16)	(14/16)	(13/16)
Bifidobacterium spp.	9.87±0.13	9.96±0.16	10.01±0.08	10.04±0.12
	(16/16)	(16/16)	(16/16)	(16/16)
Veillonella spp.	6.65±0.46	5.99±0.43	6.23±0.45	7.03±0.41
	(14/16)	(13/16)	(14/16)	(10/16)
Megashaera spp.	5.83±0.69	6.50±0.42	6.90±0.60	6.00±0.62
	(3/16)	(3/16)	(2/16)	(3/16)
Curved rods	0	0	0	0
	(0/16)	(0/16)	(0/16)	(0/16)
Clostridium spp.	8.89±0.22	8.27±0.24	7.74±0.43	8.50±0.34
	(16/16)	(16/16)	(12/16)	(16/16)
C. perfringens	5.81±0.67	5.06±0.61	4.36±0.51	5.62±0.38
	(12/16)	(8/16)	(5/16)	(11/16)
Lactobacillus spp.	5.16±0.39	4.98±0.52	4.96±0.32	4.75±0.39
	(12/16)	(11/16)	(14/16)	(16/16)
Enterobacteriaceae	8.49±0.25	8.55±0.27	8.66±0.20	8.62±0.24
	(16/16)	(16/16)	(16/16)	(16/16)
Streptococcaceae	7.75±0.27	7.63±0.19	7.52±0.21	7.91±0.25
	(16/16)	(16/16)	(16/16)	(16/16)
Micrococcaceae	2.94±0.19	3.01±0.22	4.54±0.56	3.07±0.14
	(10/16)	(9/16)	(10/16)	(9/16)
Bacillus spp.	2.93±0.20	4.45±2.15	2.53±0.11	2.85±0.25
	(3/16)	(2/16)	(6/16)	(2/16)
P. aeruginosa	3.63±0.70	3.30±0.23	3.32±0.33	3.34±0.24
	(6/16)	(8/16)	(6/16)	(11/16)
Corynebacterium spp.	3.58±0.34	3.53±0.28	3.13±0.27	3.62±0.27
	(6/16)	(4/16)	(4/16)	(6/16)
Yeasts	3.39±0.25	3.28±0.30	4.03±0.43	3.27±0.32
	(12/16)	(10/16)	(12/16)	(12/16)
Molds	0	0	0	0
	(0/16)	(0/16)	(0/16)	(0/16)

[1] Mean±S.E. of log10 bacterial cells/gram of wet feces, with occurrence frequency (number in bracket indicates the number of feces in which the bacterium indicated was observed/total samples).

[2] Means of counts and frequency of occurrence of each bacterium in Control A, Test 1, Test 2, and Control B were compared. Means having at least a similar letter were not significantly different at $p<0.05$.
Reproduced from Okubo et al. (1992) [23] by permission of the Japan Society for Bioscience, Biotechnology, and Agrochemistry, Tokyo.

Of the eighteen intestinal bacteria inspected, only clostridia bacilli were remarkably reduced by the tea polyphenols intake. The decrease in their cellular counts was observed in Test 1 and Test 2. This fact indicates that at least four weeks of continuous intake of green tea extract was necessary for causing reduction of the clostridia cell counts. Of other bacteria, *Bifidobacterium* spp. increased and Peptococcaceae decreased, but the degrees were not so significant. All other bacteria examined such as Bacteroidaceae, *Eubacterium, Veillonella, Megasphaera,* curved rods, *Lactobacillus*, enterobacteria, streptococci, micrococci, *Bacillus, Pseudomonas aeruginosa,* and *Corynebacterium* were not affected by tea polyphenols intake.

The occurrence frequency of *C. perfringens* (Table 3) was found to decrease during the test period from 12 (Control period A) to 8 (Test period 1) or to 5 of 16 samples (Test period 2) by intake of tea polyphenols. This effect of tea polyphenols was significant when the intake was continued for four weeks. However, the effect on *Clostridium* spp. was reversible, as can be seen from the result that the score of Control period B was the same as Control period A. This fact proves that tea polyphenols act as a negative adaptogen and thus, in order to keep low levels of the bacterial cell counts and their occurrence frequency, it is necessary to continue the intake of tea polyphenols as long as possible.

Table 4

Bacteria Found in Feces

Microorganisms	Control A	Test 1	Test 2	Control B
Bacteroidaceae	47.7	46.5	47.6	49.3
Eubacterium spp.	27.9	29.4	30.6	26.6
Peptococcaceae	9.9	6.9	4.6	3.9
Bifidobacterium spp.	10.2	14.2	14.8	16
Clostridium spp.[1]	2	0.8	0.5	1.8
Others[2]	2.8	2.3	2.1	2.6

[1] *C. perfringens* excluded.

[2] *Veillonella* spp., *Megasphaera* spp., *Clostridium perfringens, Lactobacillus* spp., Enterobacteriaceae, Streptococcaceae, Micrococcaceae, *Bacillus* spp., *Pseudomonas aeruginosa, Corynebacterium* spp., yeasts, and molds.

Reproduced from Okubo et al. (1992) [23] by permission of the Japan Society for Bioscience, Biotechnology, and Agrochemistry, Tokyo.

Table 4 shows the percentage composition of each bacterium of the total bacterial cell counts. *Clostridium* spp. and *Peptococcaceae* decreased in percentage during the tea polyphenol intake period and upon discontinuing the intake; the value of *Clostridium* spp. returned to that at the beginning of the test. The value of Peptococcaceae decreased continuously while *Bifidobacterium* spp. increased with intake of tea polyphenol. This is evidence that intestinal clostridia including *C. perfringens* are sensitive to tea polyphenol. Intestinal clostridia have been related with several diseases as described above.

Intestinal microflora of the patients with colon cancer have been reported to show a high percent composition of clostridia and a low percent of bifidobacteria. The tea polyphenols which were proven to selectively inhibit the growth of clostridia while promoting the growth of bifidobacteria, may be useful for controlling the bacterial balance in our large intestine. This result coincides with that obtained with an *in vitro* test in which the growth of *Clostridium* spp. was inhibited while that of *Bifidobacterium* spp. was promoted by the green tea extract.

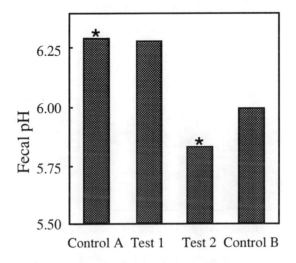

Figure 1. Effect of tea polyphenols intake on fecal pH.
*Difference is significant at $p < 0.05$ for Control A and Test 2.
Reproduced from Okubo et al. (1992) [23] by permission of the Japan Society for Bioscience, Biotechnology, and Agrochemistry, Tokyo.

As shown in Figure 1, tea polyphenols intake also resulted in a decrease of the pH value of feces. This effect may be attributed to an increase in the formation of volatile fatty acids (acetic and propionic acid, see Figure 2). As for the occurrence of putrefaction and enzyme activities of feces, however, no significant difference was observed between the volunteers' feces with and without tea polyphenols (Figures 3 and 4; Table 5). But, by intake of tea polyphenols, the pH value of intestine was stabilized at a low level. This result will serve to improve the intestinal condition to reduce formation of harmful bacterial metabolism [24]. The increase in the percentage composition of *Bifidobacterium* spp. (acid forming bacteria) is thought, of course, to be a cause of pH reduction. The increase in formation of volatile fatty acids was found to be proportional with the increase in the percentage composition of the acid forming bacteria, mainly of *Bifidobacteriuum* spp. The acids are also causal compounds to decrease pH value. Several putrefactive products and enzymes which are known to be associated with several diseases were also investigated [25]. However, those parameters were not found to change even when tea polyphenols intake was continued. The odor of feces excreted during tea polyphenols intake clearly became less than those obtained during the control periods. The odor seemed to consist of mainly indole, skatole, cresol, and ammonia. The amounts of those compounds may have been decreased by reaction with certain component(s) of tea polyphenols administered. The quantity of tea polyphenols given to the volunteers daily was slightly more than that contained in 10 cups of green tea infusion usually served as a drink a day. In spite of intake of relatively large amounts of tea polyphenols for four weeks, no undesirable or abnormal effects were observed for the volunteers. The result of blood analysis of the volunteers also showed that the intake of tea polyphenols did not bring any effect on their metabolism (Table 6) [26].

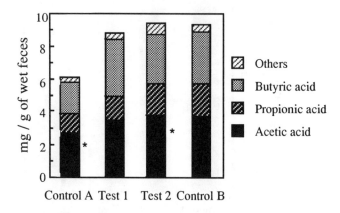

Figure 2. Effects of tea polyphenols intake on fecal volatile fatty acids.
*Difference is significant at $p < 0.05$ for Control A and Test 2.
Others includes valeric and caproic acids.
Reproduced from Okubo et al. (1992) [23] by permission of the Japan Society for Bioscience, Biotechnology, and Agrochemistry, Tokyo.

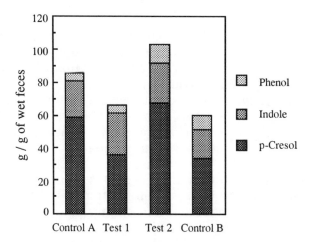

Figure 3. Effects of tea polyphenols intake on fecal putrefactive products.
Minor components such as skatol and 4-ethylphenol are not shown here.
Reproduced from Okubo et al. (1992) [23] by permission of the Japan Society for Bioscience, Biotechnology, and Agrochemistry, Tokyo.

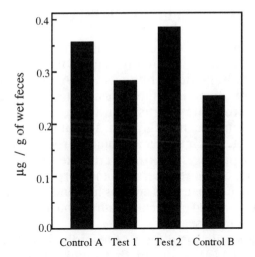

Figure 4. Effects of tea polyphenols intake on fecal ammonia content. Reproduced from Okubo et al. (1992) [23] by permission of the Japan Society for Bioscience, Biotechnology, and Agrochemistry, Tokyo.

Table 5

Effects of Tea Polyphenols Intake on Some Enzyme Activities of Feces

	Control A	Test 1	Test 2	Control B
β-Glucosidase	57.49±35.14	61.50±39.61	65.86±55.96	49.15±22.34
β-Glucuronidase	30.53±19.72	34.75±18.88	40.50±27.06	37.13±25.72
Nitroreductase	6.31±3.09	7.44±2.85	7.98±3.50	6.94±4.69

Values are means ± S.D. (μmol/g/hr).
Reproduced from Okubo et al. (1992) [23] by permission of the Japan Society for Bioscience, Biotechnology, and Agrochemistry, Tokyo.

Table 6

Effects of Tea Polyphenols Intake on Some Blood Components

Compounds, mg/dl	Control A	Test 1	Test 2	Control B
Total cholesterol	192±29	182±28	180±32	184±37
Free cholesterol	51.8±8.0	47.8±8.2	46.9±8.6**	47.9±10.2
Ester ratio	72.5±0.9	73.3±0.9*	73.7±1.0	73.7±0.8**
β-lipoprotein	358±52	368±108	330±58	340±72
HDL-cholesterol	57.0±11.3	59.4±12.9	55.1±12.0	55.5±11.9

Values are means ± S.D.
Difference is significant at $p<0.01$** and $p<0.05$*.
Reproduced from Okubo et al. (1991) [26] by permission of Proceeding of the International Symposium on Tea Science, Shizuoka.

IV. ANTIVIRAL EFFECT OF TEA POLYPHENOLS

Viruses contain either DNA or RNA, but both are not found in one virus. Hepadna virus, popova virus, adenovirus, herpes virus, poxvirus and parvovirus are DNA viruses pathogenic to humans. RNA viruses are picornavirus, enterovirus, calicivirus, togavirus, flavivirus, orthomyxovirus, paramyxovirus, coronavirus, arenavirus, bunyavirus, retrovirus, rhabdovirus, and reovirus. These viruses infect humans through skin, sexual organs, respiratory organs, and digestive tracts when their tissues are injured. The general symptoms caused by establishment of pathogenic viruses are toxemia, fever, weakness, and diminishing appetite. Some retroviruses and herpesviruses are known to be carcinogenic. The countermeasures such as hygiene, sanitation, vector control, vaccination, and physical and chemical treatment have been taken for protection from occurrence of viral disease.

This section deals with the effects of tea polyphenols against these viral infections. Green (1949) reported that black tea extract inhibited the multiplication of influenza A virus in embryonated eggs [27]. The extract of green tea leaves has also been reported to show antiviral activity against influenza virus [28], vaccinia virus, herpes simplex virus, Coxsackie virus B6, and poliovirus 1 [29]. Mukoyama and his colleagues reported with an *in vitro* test that (-)-epigallocatechin gallate (EGCg) from green tea and teaflavin digallate (TF3) from black tea blocked the infectivity of both rotavirus and enterovirus in cultured rhesus monkey kidney MA 104 cells [30] and influenza A and B virus in Madin-Darby canine kidney (MDCK) cells [31]. Also, they observed that EGCg and TF3 inhibited the haemagglutination activity of the influenza virus. These findings suggested that EGCg or TF3 binds haemagglutinin of the influenza virus and that the adsorption onto MDCK cells of the virus become unattainable. Influenza is a disease with a high mortality rate and occasionally spreads throughout the world.

We examined the effect of green tea polyphenols on rotavirus [32, 33]. Rotaviruses belonging to the Reoviridae family are causal viruses of gastroenteritis which sometimes happens in infants and children [34, 35]. Although diarrheal diseases are among the most common illness, several millions of infants and children have been reported to suffer from diarrhea in the world annually, and about half of the cases have been caused by viruses including rotavirus.

We observed that the tea polyphenols strongly inhibit the propagation of rotavirus cultured in rhesus monkey kidney MA 104 cells. As shown in Table 7, (-)-epicatechin gallate and (-)-epigallocatechin gallate were strongly effective and, at a concentration of 1 mg/ml, they inhibited the propagation by 84.4% and 96.2%, respectively. Gallic acid and its derivatives were not effective. These results suggested that the galloyl moiety linked by ester linkage in catechin molecule is important for the antivirus activity.

In China, green tea has been applied to the treatment of diarrhea. This fact is a suggestion that a certain component(s) of green tea is effective for prevention from or treatment of diarrhea caused by rotavirus or/and bacteria. Ono and his colleagues reported that certain tea polyphenols and several other flavonoids were strong inhibitors of reverse transcriptase of HIV (human immunodeficiency virus) and several DNA- and RNA-polymerases [36, 37].

HIV is a retrovirus, and its reverse transcriptase is important for HIV establishment in the host cells. ECg and EGCg were found to be strong inhibitors of HIV-reverse transcriptase, whereas EC, EGC, and gallic acid were ineffective. The concentration of ECg and EGCg for a 50% inhibition of HIV-reverse transcriptase were only 0.017 mg/ml and 0.012 mg/ml, respectively. It is highly likely that the effective polyphenols mentioned above will be developed to apply for prevention from or treatment of various diseases due to viruses.

Table 7

Antivirus Effect of Tea

Polyphenols on Human Rotavirus

Green Tea Polyphenols*	Inhibition (%)
(+)-Catechin	25.7
(-)-Epicatechin	7.3
(+)-Gallocatechin	not tested
(-)-Epicatechin gallate	84.4
(-)-Epigallocatechin	37.6
(-)-Epigallocatechin gallate	96.2

*Concentration of polyphenols applied was 1µg/ml.
Reproduced from Ebina (1991) [33] by permission of the Society for Antibacterial and Antifungal Agents, Japan.

REFERENCES

1. **Hentges, D. J.,** Role of the intestinal microflora in host defense against infection, in *Human Intestinal Microflora in Health and Disease*, Hentges, D. J., Ed., Academic Press, New York, 1983, p 311.
2. **Mitsuoka, T.,** *A Color Atlas of Anaerobic Bacteria*, Shobunsha, Tokyo, 1984.
3. **Bokkenheuser, V. D.,** Biotransformation of steroids, in *Human Intestinal Microflora in Health and Disease*, Hentges, D. J., Ed., Academic Press, New York, 1983, p 215.
4. **Goldman, P.,** Biochemical pharmacology and toxicology involving the intestinal flora, in *Human Intestinal Microflora in Health and Disease*, Hentges, D. J., Ed., Academic Press, New York, 1983, p 241.
5. **Gary, L. S. and Sherwood, L. G.,** Intestinal flora in health and disease, *Gastroenterlogy*, **86**, 174, 1984.
6. **McCarthy, R. E. and Salyers, A. A.,** The effects of dietary fiber utilization on the colonic microflora, in *Human Intestinal Microflora in Health and Disease*, Hentges, D. J., Ed., Academic Press, New York, 1983, p 295.

7. **Salyers, A. A. and Leedle, J. A. Z.,** Carbohydrate metabolism in the human colon, in *Role of the Gut Flora in Toxicity and Cancer,* Academic Press, New York, 1988, p 129.
8. **Rowland, I. R., Mallett, A. K., and Wise, A.,** The effect of diet on the mammalian gut flora and its metabolic activities, in *CRC Critical Reviews in Toxicology,* **Vol. 16,** CRC Press, Inc., 1985, p 31.
9. **Ahn, Y. J., Kim, M., Yamamoto, T., Fujisawa, T., and Mitsuoka, T.,** Selective growth responses of human intestinal bacteria to Araliaceae plant extracts, *Microb. Ecol. in Health and Disease,* 3, 169, 1990.
10. **Ahn, Y. J., Sakanaka, S., Kim, M., Kawamura, T., Fujisawa, T., and Mitsuoka, T.,** Effect of green tea extract on growth of intestinal bacteria, *Microb. Ecol. in Health and Disease,* 3, 335, 1990.
11. **Ahn, A. J., Kawamura, T., Kim, M., Yamamoto, T., and Mitsuoka, T.,** The polyphenols: selective growth inhibitors of *Clostridium* spp., *Agric. Biol. Chem.,* **55,** 1425, 1991.
12. **Kada, T., Kaneko, K., Matsuzaki, T., and Hara, Y.,** Detection and chemical identification of natural bio-antimutagens. A case of the green tea factor, *Mutat. Res.,* **150,** 127, 1985.
13. **Weisburger, J. H., Nagano, M., Wakabayashi, K., and Oguri, A.,** Prevention of heterocyclic amine formation by tea and tea polyphenols, *Cancer Lett.,* **83,** 143, 1994.
14. **Okuda, T., Kimura, Y., Yoshida, T., Hatano, T., Okuda, H., and Arichi, S.,** Studies on the activities of tannins and related compounds from medical plants and drugs. I. Inhibitory effects on lipid peroxidation in mitochondria and microsomes of liver, *Chemical and Pharmaceutical Bulletin,* **31,** 1625, 1983.
15. **Hara, Y., Nakamura, K., Fujino, R., Hosaka, H., Kohisae, S., Asai, H., and Sugiura, M.,** Antitumor action of the green tea extract, *Proceedings of Annual Meeting Japanese Society of Cancer Research, Nagoya,* 1984, p 993.
16. **Yamane, T., Hagiwara, N., Tateishi, M., Akachi, S., Kim, M., Okuzumi, J., Kitao, Y., Inagake, M., Kuwata, K., and Takahashi, T.,** Inhibition of azoxymethane-induced colon carcinogenesis in rat by green tea polyphenol fraction, *Jpn. J. Cancer Res.,* **82,** 1336, 1991.
17. **Yamane, T., Takahashi, T., Kuwata, K., Oya, K., Inagake, M., Kitao, Y., Suganuma, M., and Fujiki, H.,** Inhibition of N-Methyl-N'-nitro-N-nitrosoguanidine-induced carcinogenesis by (-)-epigallocatechin gallate in the rat glandular stomach, *Cancer Res.,* **55,** 2081, 1995.
18. **Yamane, T., Inagake, M., Kimuoka, M., Matsumoto, M., Oya, K., Takahashi, T., and Fujiki, H.,** Cancer chemoprevention with green tea extract, in *Proceedings of Annual Meeting Japanese Society of Cancer Research, Nagoya,* 1994, p 117.
19. **Matsuzaki, T. and Hara, Y.,** Antioxidative activity of tea leaf catechins, *Nippon Nogeikagaku Kaishi,* **59,** 124, 1985.
20. **Sakanaka, S., Kim, M., Taniguchi, M., and Yamamoto, T.,** Antibacterial substances in Japanese green tea extract against *Streptococcus mutans,* a cariogenic bacterium, *Agric. Biol. Chem.,* **53,** 2307, 1989.
21. **Toda, M., Okubo, S., Hiyoshi, R., and Shimamura, T.,** The bacterial activity of tea and coffee, *Lett. Appl. Microbiol.,* **8,** 123, 1989.

22. **Kakuda, T., Matsuura, T., Mortelmans, K., and Parkhurst, R.,** Biological activity of tea extracts on Bifidobacterium proliferation, in *Proceedings of the International Symposium on Tea Science,* Kurofune Printing Co. Ltd., Shizuoka, 1991, p 357.
23. **Okubo, T., Ishihara, N., Oura, A., Serit, M., Kim, M., Yamamoto, T., and Mitsuoka, T.,** *In vivo* effects of tea polyphenols intake on human intestinal microflora and metabolisms, *Biosci. Biotech. Biochem.,* **56**, 588, 1992.
24. **Pietroiusti, A., Caprilli, R., Giuliano, M., Serrano, S., and Vita, S.,** Faecal pH in colorectal cancer, *Ital. J. Gastroenterol.,* **17**, 88, 1985.
25. **Kinoshita, N. and Gelboin, H. V.,** β-glucronidase catalyzed hydrolysis of benzo (a) pyrene-3-glucuronide and binding to DNA, *Science,* **199**, 307, 1978.
26. **Okubo, T., Ishihara, N., Oura, A., and Kim, M.,** Effect of tea polyphenol intake on intestinal microflora and metabolism, in *Proceedings of the International Symposium on Tea Science,* Kurofune Printing Co. Ltd., Shizuoka, 1991, p 299.
27. **Green, R. H.,** Inhibition of multiplication of influenza virus by extracts of tea, *Proc. Soc. Exp. Biol. Med.,* **71**, 84, 1949.
28. **Nakayama, M., Toda, M., Okubo, S., and Shimamura, T.,** Inhibition of influenza virus infection by tea, *Lett. Appl. Microbiol.,* **11**, 38, 1990.
29. **John, T. J. and Mukundan, P.,** Virus inhibition by tea, caffeine and tannic acid, *Ind. J. Med. Res.,* **69**, 542, 1979.
30. **Mukoyama, A., Ushijima, H., Nishimura, S., Koike, H., Toda, M., Hara, Y., and Shimamura, T.,** Inhibition of rotavirus and enterovirus infections by tea extracts, *Jpn. J. Med. Sci. Biol.,* **44**, 181, 1991.
31. **Nakayama, M., Suzuki, K., Toda, M., Okubo, S., Hara, Y., and Shimamura, T.,** Inhibition of the infectivity of influenza virus by tea polyphenols, *Antivir. Res.,* **21**, 289, 1993.
32. **Hatta, H., Sakanaka, S., Tsuda, N., Kim, M., Yamamoto, T., and Ebina, T.,** Anti-infectious substances in green tea against rotavirus, in *37th Annual Meeting of Japanese Society of Virologists, Osaka,* 1989, 327.
33. **Ebina, T.,** Infantile gastroenteritis: prevention and treatment of rotaviral diarrhea., *J. Antibact. Antifung. Agents,* **19**, 349, 1991.
34. **Barnett, B.,** Viral gastroenteritis, *Med. Clin. N. Am.,* **67**, 1031, 1983.
35. **Cukor, G. and Blacklow, N. R.,** Human viral gastroenteritis, *Microbiol. Rev.,* **48**, 157, 1984.
36. **Ono, K. and Nakane, H.,** Catechins as a novel class of inhibitors for HIV-reverse transcriptase and DNA polymerases, in *Proceedings of the International Symposium on Tea Science,* Kurofune Printing Co. Ltd., Shizuoka, 1991, p 277.
37. **Nakane, H. and Ono, K.,** Differential inhibitory effects of some catechin derivatives on the activities of human immunodeficiency virus reverse transcriptase and cellular deoxyribonucleic and ribonucleic acid polymerases, *Biochemistry,* **29**, 2841, 1990.

Chapter 11

DEODORIZING EFFECT OF GREEN TEA EXTRACTS

M. Hibino and S. Sakanaka

TABLE OF CONTENTS

I. Introduction
II. Deodorizing Effect of Green Tea Polyphenols
    A. Effect on Methyl Mercaptan
    B. Effect on Trimethylamine
    C. Effect on Ammonia
    D. Effect on Tobacco Smoke
III. Applications of Green Tea Extracts as a Deodorant
References

I. INTRODUCTION

Many people mind unpleasant odors or reeks generated from things such as tobacco, garlic, fish, feces, etc. that often occur in our daily life. The deodorizing effect of green tea leaves has been known from old time, and tea leaves have been traditionally used as a deodorant material [1]. In Japan, people usually drink green tea infusion with or after taking a meal. Drinking green tea infusion is also known to neutralize the foul breath occasionally generated depending on the kind of meal. This deodorant effect is thought to be attributed to polyphenolic compounds contained in green tea infusion. The content of polyphenolic compounds in green tea leaves amounts to 10-15%, and most of them are so-called tea polyphenols such as (+)-catechin, (-)-epicatechin, (+)-gallocatechin, (-)-epigallocatechin, (-)-epicatechin gallate, and (-)-epigallocatechin gallate [2]. Recently, Yasuda and Arakawa reported on the deodorizing action of green tea in the test against methyl mercaptan that among tea polyphenols, EGCg showed the strongest deodorizing action. They suggested that the deodorizing action of EGCg against methyl mercaptan is by the reactivity of -OH groups on B ring of EGCg which change into orthoquinone type by exposure to air and conjugate with a thiomethyl or methyl sulfinyl group resulting in a thioether or sulfinyl ether [3].

The present chapter deals with the deodorizing action of green tea extract against various odors or reeks which are often present in our surroundings.

II. DEODORIZING EFFECT OF GREEN TEA POLYPHENOLS

Green tea extract prepared according to the method described in Chapter 13 contains several polyphenolic compounds. They are derivatives of catechin, and the hydroxyl groups of the polyphenols (see Chapters 3 and 4) are known to be reactive with thiol or amino (ammonium) groups.

Nasty odors we often smell in our surroundings are usually a mixture of several compounds, for example, the odor of halitosis consists of methyl mercaptan, hydrogen sulfide, dimethyl sulfide, etc., which are produced in the breakdown of proteins by bacteria or enzymes in tissues [4, 5]. Among these compounds, methyl mercaptan is most closely related with halitosis [6]. Also, most of the bad smells produced in uncontrolled or neglected foods or in waste foods are of amide compounds.

We examined the effect of green tea extract (Sunflavon[R], Taiyo Kagaku Co., Ltd.) on methyl mercaptan, trimethylamine, and ammonia as typical bad smell compounds [7]. The general composition of green tea extract used here was as follows: polyphenols 30%; reducing sugar as glucose 14%; total sugar content, 30.5%; amino acids as glutamic acid, 2.6%; ash, 9.8%; and moisture, 3.8%.

A. EFFECT ON METHYL MERCAPTAN

Methyl mercaptan is a typical bad smelling compound generated in our mouths. Several plant extracts have been investigated for their deodorizing activities against methyl mercaptan [8-10], and the effect of green tea polyphenols was found to be pronounced on analysis with gas chromatography. The effect was evaluated to be superior to sodium copper chlorophyllin which has been used as a deodorizer.

The analysis of deodorizing activities was carried out by the following method: 1 ml of 0.3% sodium methyl mercaptan solution to 1 ml of 0.1% or 0.5% green tea extract solution placed in a 10 ml glass vial was added. The vial was then captured and allowed to stand at 37°C for 5 min, and the head space air was taken for analysis with gas chromatography.

The deodorant activity of the green tea extract against methyl mercaptan was stronger than that of sodium copper chlorophyllin (Table 1).

Table 1
Effect of Green Tea Extract as
a Deodorant against Methyl Mercaptan and Trimethylamine*

Compound examined	Decrease in head space air, %		
	Deodorant		
	Green tea extract		SCC**
	0.1%	0.5%	0.2%
Methyl mercaptan	87.4	94.0	42.1
Trimethylamine	84.4	89.6	83.0

*See the text.
** Sodium copper chrolophyllin
Gas chromatographic conditions: Shimadzu gas chromatography GC-9A; column, SUPELCOWAX 10, 30 m x 0.25 mm ID, 0.25 μm film; carrier, N_2 1 ml/min; Inj., split (50:1), 200°C; sample applied, 1 ml head-space air; oven, 60°C; detector, FID.

B. EFFECT ON TRIMETHYLAMINE

Trimethylamine is a major compound which wards off smells produced in "reserved fish" or "fish shop smell." The effect of green tea extract on trimethylamine was examined by the same method as done for methyl mercaptan, and it was found to be effective for removal of the odor of trimethylamine (Table 1). Hatae and her colleagues reported that the amount of amines analyzed by gas chromatography of the fish cooked in tea extract solution was less than that cooked in tap water [11].

C. EFFECT ON AMMONIA

Ammonia is also a stinking compound and its trace amount affects the quality of various foods or other articles. The deodorizing effect of green tea extract on ammonia was examined by the following method: 1 ml of 0.2% or 1.0% solution of green tea extract was made to penetrate into a piece of adsorbent cotton (3 x 3 cm, 0.15 g) and placed in a 3 l volume plastic bottle. On one hand, ammonia solution (25%) was stored at 37°C, and 1 ml of the head-space air of the container was taken with a syringe and administered into the plastic bottle. After standing for 5 min at room temperature, the concentration of ammonia in the air inside the plastic bottle was determined by using an ammonia gas detector system (Gastec Corp., Japan).

The concentration of ammonia gas was distinctly decreased by the presence of adsorbent cotton wetted with a solution of green tea extract (Table 2).

Table 2

Effect of Green Tea Extract as a Deodorant toward Ammonia and Tobacco Smoke*

Compound examined	Decrease in head space air, %		
	Deodorant		
	Green tea extract		SCC**
	0.1%	0.5%	0.2%
Methyl mercaptan	87.4	94.0	42.1
Trimethylamine	84.4	89.6	83.0

*See the text.

** Sodium copper chrolophyllin

Gas chromatographic conditions: Shimadzu gas chromatography GC-9A; column, SUPELCOWAX 10, 30 m x 0.25 mm ID, 0.25 μm film; carrier, N_2 1 ml/min; Inj., split (50:1), 200°C; sample applied, 1 ml head-space air; oven, 60°C; detector, FID.

D. EFFECT ON TOBACCO SMOKE

The smell of smoking tobacco is also generally hated and hazardous. This is particularly true in a small room, because the smell is retained for a while. Recently, it is said that tobacco smoke contains cancer causing compounds. One ml of 0.2% or 1.0% solution of the green tea extract was placed in a 10 ml glass vial, and after administration of 1 ml of tobacco smoke to the bottom of the air space of the vial using a syringe, the vial was capped and incubated at

37°C. After 5 min of incubation, the head-space gas was analyzed by gas chromatography. A deeodorizing effect was expressed by the decreasing ratio of the main peaks of the gas chromatogram.

The result revealed that the green tea extract showed a distinct effect, deodorizing the smoking smell, and that the effect was superior compared to sodium copper chlorophyllin examined under the same conditions (Table 2).

III. APPLICATIONS OF GREEN TEA EXTRACTS AS DEODORANT

Candies were prepared with green tea extract (1 mg green tea extract per g), and their deodorizing effect was examined for the smell remaining in the mouth after eating garlic. Several volunteers gargled with an extract of mashed garlic, and their breaths were immediately collected into a plastic bag. Then, the volunteers put a piece of the candy (3.3 g) in their mouths for 4 min and finally swallowed it. Their breaths were collected, and the halitosis before and after eating the candy were subjected to the sensory test. The appraisal was graded from 0 to 4 as follows: 0, very strong smell; 1, strong smell; 2, medium smell; 3, weak smell; and 4, no smell. The deodorizing effect was expressed by the mean value of this score.

Upon licking the candy containing green tea extract, the halitosis of volunteers was definitely reduced (Table 3). A similar result was also obtained by oolong tea which also contained polyphenols. Yasuda and his coworkers investigated the effect of chewing gum added with green tea extract for halitosis, and they confirmed the deodorizing effect [12].

The preparation of green tea polyphenols was also found to be effective as a deodorant for smell generated during the processing of fish and various animal meat products [13].

The elucidation of the mechanism involved in the deodorizing activity of green tea polyphenols is under study now, and its dissolution will bring a wide application of green tea polyphenols as a deodorant in various fields of industry and our daily home life.

Table 3
Deodorizing Effect of Candies
Containing Green Tea Extract on the Garlic Odor*

Additions*	Appraisal of the breath***
None (Control)	1.3
Green tea extract 0.1%	3.7
SCC** 0.1%	1.3

*See the text.
**Sodium copper chrolophyllin.

***Examined by four pannel members.

REFERENCES

1. **Kubokawa, Y. and Fukushima, K.,** Cha no Daijiten (in Japanese), in *Cha no Daijiten*, "Ocha no Daijiten" Kankoukai, Shizuoka, 1991, p 322.
2. **Sakanaka, S., Kim, M., Taniguchi, M., and Yamamoto, T.,** Antibacterial substances in Japanese green tea extract against *Streptococcus mutans*, a cariogenic bacterium, *Agric. Biol. Chem.*, **53**, 2307, 1989.
3. **Yasuda, H. and Arakawa, T.,** Deodorizing mechanism of (-)-epigallocatechin gallate against methyl mercaptan, *Biosci. Biotech. Biochem.*, **59**, 1232, 1995.
4. **Kaizu, T.,** Analysis of volatile sulphur compounds in mouth air by gas chromatography, *Nippon Shishubyo Gakkaishi (in Japanese)*, **18**, 1, 1976.
5. **Richter, V. J. and Tonzetich, J.,** The application of instrumental technique for the evaluation of odoriferous volatiles from saliva and breath, *Arch. Oral Biol.*, **9**, 47, 1964.
6. **Kaizu, T., Tsunoda, M., Aoki, H., and Kimura, K.,** Analysis of volatile sulphur compounds in mouth air by gas chromatography, *Bull. Tokyo Dent. Coll.*, **19**, 43, 1978.
7. **Aizawa, M. and Nakamura, I.,** Application of deodorizing components in green tea, *Shokuhin to Kaihatsu (in Japanese)*, **27**, 43, 1992.
8. **Tokita, F., Ishikawa, M., and Shibuya, K.,** Deodorizing activity of some plant extracts against methyl mercaptan, *Nippon Nogeikagaku Kaishi (in Japanese)*, **58**, 585, 1984.
9. **Nakatani, N., Miura, K., and Inagaki, T.,** Structure of new deodorant biphenyl compounds from thyme (*Thymus vulgaris* L.) and their activity against methyl mercaptan, *Agric. Biol. Chem.*, **53**, 1375, 1989.
10. **Yasuda, H. and Ui, M.,** Deodorant effect of plant extracts of the family Rosaceae against methyl mercaptan, *Nippon Nogeikagaku Kaishi (in Japanese)*, **66**, 1475, 1992.
11. **Hatae, K., Sato, T., and Yoshimatsu, F.,** Effect of green tea infusions on tenderness of bones and intensity of odors in cooked fish, *Kaseigaku Zasshi (in Japanese)*, **31**, 88, 1980.
12. **Yasuda, H., Moriyama, T., and Tsunoda, M.,** The effect of chewing gum for halitosis by gas chromatograph (III) Investigation for chewing gum containing tea extracts, *Nippon Shishubyo Gakkai Kaishi (in Japanese)*, **37**, 141, 1995.
13. **Dohi, S., Motosugi, M., Suzuki, K., and Hamajima, T.,** Utilization of tea leaf (II) Test production of a new food stuff with tea leaf paste, *Shizuokaken Shizuoka Kogyo Gijutsu Center Kenkyu Hokoku (in Japanese)*, **35**, 70, 1990.

Chapter 12

THEANINE - ITS SYNTHESIS, ISOLATION, AND PHYSIOLOGICAL ACTIVITY

D.-C. Chu, K. Kobayashi, L. R. Juneja, and T. Yamamoto

TABLE OF CONTENTS

I. Introduction
II. Biosynthesis of Theanine and Its Metabolism in Tea Plant
III. Enzymic Synthesis of Theanine
IV. Physiological Activity of Theanine
References

I. INTRODUCTION

Theanine is a unique amino acid because it is found only in tea plant with the exception of mushroom and seedlings of a few kinds of *Camellia species, C. japonica* and *C. sasanqua*. Theanine in tea leaf accounts for about 50% of all free amino acids. The occurrence of theanine in tea leaves was discovered by Sakato in 1950, and its chemical structure was determined to be γ-ethylamino-L-glutamic acid [1]. Casimir and his colleagues (1960) isolated a derivative of glutamic acid from the nonprotein nitrogen fraction of the mushroom *Xerocomus badius*. They identified the derivative to be N'-ethyl-γ-glutamine (theanine) by paper chromatography and other analytical methods [2]. Theanine as well as glutamine has been known to act antagonistically against paralysis induced by caffeine. Also, several chemical derivatives including theanine and γ-aminobutyric acid found in green tea have been reported to be physiologically active substances in various animals and plants [3, 4].

Tea leaf is a sole natural resource of theanine reported to present. However, recently the production of theanine has become possible to be carried out in an industrial scale by the method of enzymic synthesis. It was also found that the intake of theanine brings the generation of α-brain waves in humans.

Theanine is also one of the components that decides its taste (umami). This chapter deals with theanine presence in tea plant, its enzymic synthesis, and some of its physiological activities.

II. BIOSYNTHESIS OF THEANINE AND ITS METABOLISM IN TEA PLANT

The ammonium assimilation pattern of tea plants is characteristic. Theanine is synthesized in the root starting from ammonium as the nitrogen source [5]. The glutamic acid produced in the root conjugates with ethylamine by the catalytic reaction of L-glutamate ethylamine ligase (E.C.,6.3.1.6) [6]. Ethylamine is derived from alanine by decarboxylation or denovo synthesis via pyruvic acid. It is known that *Camellia sinensis* produces ethylamine from alanine [7].

Theanine synthesized in the root is immediately transferred to growing shoots and accumulated there. A remarkable accumulation of theanine in buds and young leaves is due to the continuous transport of it from roots, because the catabolism of theanine in young shoots is slow relative to the transportation rate of theanine [8].

Theanine accumulated in young shoots is hydrolyzed into glutamic acid and ethylamine by an enzyme. The ethylamine produced is used to synthesize catechins under the sunlight [9, 10]. A part of ethylamine is degraded into acetaldehyde, hydrogen peroxide, and ammonia by an enzymic oxidation reaction. The released ammonia is used as a nitrogen source again (Figure 1). It was also revealed in an experiment using radioisotope (RI) labeled compounds that nitrogen of ethylamine is widely utilized in the synthesis of various amino acids, especially threonine and glycine. On the other hand, glutamic acid is used to produce aspartic acid and alanine under aerobic conditions, but under anaerobic conditions, it is converted into γ-aminobutyric acid and alanine by transamination reaction [11]. The amino acids generated are utilized for the synthesis of various other derivatives.

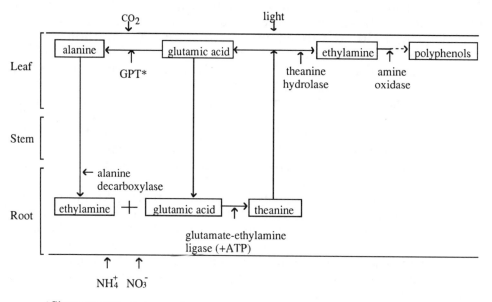

Figure 1. Schematic representation of synthesis and metabolism of theanine in tea plant [5-10].

III. ENZYMIC SYNTHESIS OF THEANINE

Theanine has been reported to have various physiological activities, and its applications in foods are being explored. Besides isolation from green tea leaves, we investigated a cost-effective method for the production and purification of theanine.

Many attempts have been made for production of theanine, however, most of them have remained unsuccessful, because of low yields, too expensive cost, highly complicated processes, etc. [12, 13, 14].

An enzymic synthetic method of theanine from glutamine and ethylamine was first reported by Yamada and his coworkers in 1990, using glutaminase from *Pseudomonas nitroreducens* [15]. Our research group also investigated the enzymic synthesis of theanine and established a practically effective method for the production of theanine on an industrial scale [16, 17].

P. nitroreducens IFO 12694 were immobilized with κ-carrageenan (Figure 2) and packed into a series of cylindrical reactors (Figure 3). Solutions of 0.3M glutamine and 0.7M ethanolamine in 0.05M borate-NaOH buffer (pH9.5) were mixed and immediately supplied to the reactor at a flow rate of SV=0.33 h^{-1} at 30°C. By this method, production of theanine was operated for over a period of 120 days with a high yield of the product (Figure 4). The theanine in the product reservoir was easily isolated by subjecting the solution to column chromatography using an ion exchanger. The yield of theanine was about 95% based on glutamine consumed.

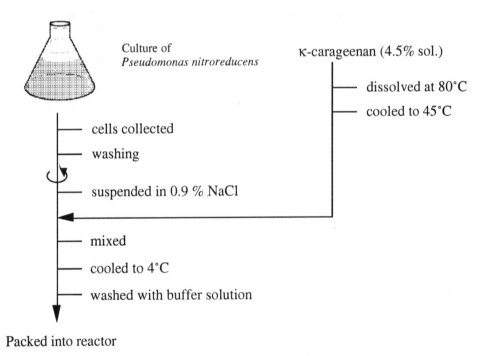

Figure 2. Preparation of immobilized cells [16, 17].

IV. PHYSIOLOGICAL ACTIVITY OF THEANINE

Theanine is known to act as an antagonist against paralysis induced by caffeine. Caffeine increases the levels of 5-hydroxytryptamine (serotonin) and 5-hydroxyindoleacetic acid. Kimura and Murata reported that theanine

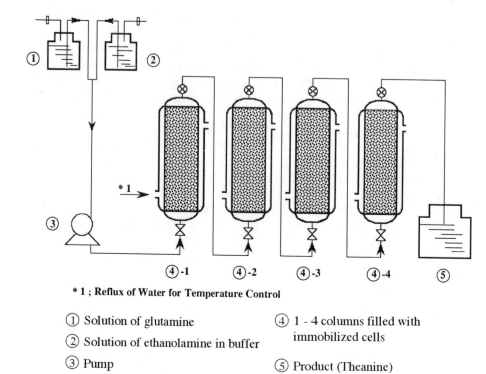

* 1 ; Reflux of Water for Temperature Control

① Solution of glutamine
② Solution of ethanolamine in buffer
③ Pump
④ 1 - 4 columns filled with immobilized cells
⑤ Product (Theanine)

Figure 3. A series of reactors for production of theanine. Reactors can be exchanged individually when activity of immobilized cell declined [16, 17].

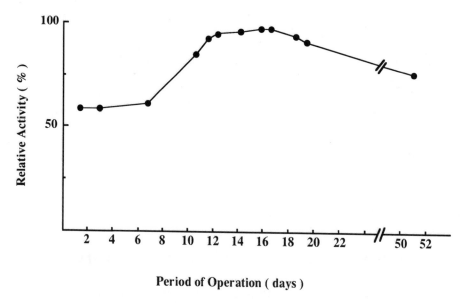

Figure 4. Relative activity of theanine synthesis by an immobilized cell reactor [16].

decreases the levels of norepinephrine and serotonin in rat brain [18]. It was found that unlike glutamine theanine of a large dosage (more than 1500 mg/kg weight) administered intraperitoneally caused significant decrease in blood pressure in spontaneously hypertensive rats [19]. It was an important finding that theanine intraperitoneally administered to rats reaches their brain in 30 min without any metabolic changes [4, 20]. Theanine administrated to rats serves the synthesis of nerve growth factor and the effect is comparable to epinephrine [21]. The meanings mentioned above are described below.

Theanine is also known to be a neurotransmitter in the brain. Yokogashi and his colleagues reported that the administration of theanine to naturally hypertensive rats resulted in a decrease in blood pressure as well as the level of 5-hydroxyindoleacetic acid in brain significantly [4]. These pharmacological and physiological effects of theanine were also demonstrated in the experiment using other animals. Our group discovered a relaxation-causing effect of theanine in human volunteers.

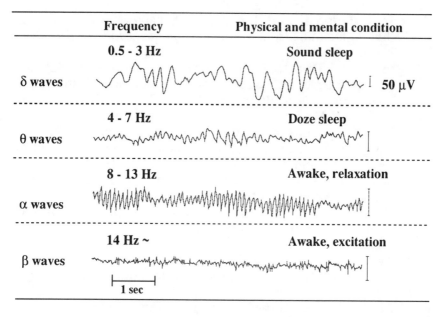

Figure 5. Classification and relation between wavelengths appearing in human brain.

In general, animals always generate a very weak electric pulse on the surface of brain, called brain waves. The frequency and amplitude of brain waves are highly related to the mental condition. The generation of a band of low frequencies in brain represents a condition leading to doze sleeps while that of high frequency, a condition of excitation (Figure 5). Plate 7 following page 36 shows a result obtained in the brain topography visualization by the computer analyzing technique when theanine was orally administered to volunteers. The α-brain waves generated were observed in a broad region of their brain surfaces within 40 min. This observation seems to be interesting and important not only in the study of the physiology of the cerebrum, but also in the development of a novel type of tranquilizer.

Theanine has been recognized as a kind of amino acid to give a specific taste to green tea infusion and as an antagonist against caffeine. In other words, theanine is a unique amino acid to show interesting physiological functions. As the industrial production of theanine has been achieved, this attractive amino acid may become a functional additive to foods to make stressed people relax. Theanine is a safe and non habit-forming substance. Therefore, it has been taken by people for thousands years as a component of green tea.

REFERENCES

1. **Sakato, Y.**, The chemical constituents of tea: III. A new amide theanine., *J. Agri. Chem. Soc.*, **23**, 262, 1950.
2. **Casimir, J., Jadot, J., and Renard, M.**, Separation and characterization of N'-ethyl-γ-glutamine from *Xerocomus badius*, *Biochim. Biophys. Acta*, **39**, 462, 1960.
3. **Kimura, R. and Murata, T.**, Influence of alkylamides of glutamic acid and related compounds on the central nervous system. I. Central depressant effect of theanine, *Chem. Pharm. Bull.*, **19**, 1257, 1971.
4. **Kimura, R. and Murata, T.**, Influence of alkylamides of glutamic acid and related compounds on the central nervous system. II. Syntheses of amides of glutamic acid and related compounds, and their effects on the central nervous system, *Chem. Pharm. Bull.*, **19**, 1301, 1971.
5. **Konishi, S. and Takahashi, E.**, Metabolism of theanine in tea seedlings and transport of the metabolites, *J. Soil and Manure*, **40**, 479, 1969.
6. **Sasaoka, K., Kito, M., and Onishi, Y.**, Some properties of the theanine synthesizing enzyme in tea seedlings, *Agric. Biol. Chem.*, **29**, 984, 1965.
7. **Takeo, T.**, L-Alanine as a precursor of ethylamine in *Camellia sinensis*, *Phytochemistry*, **13**, 1401, 1974.
8. **Takeo, T.**, Ammonium-type nitrogen assimilation in tea plants, *Agric. Biol. Chem.*, **44**, 2007, 1980.
9. **Konishi, S.**, Studies on the metabolism of theanine in tea plant using radioactive carbon. Japan Conference on Radioisotopes, in *9th Japan Atomic Industry Forum,* 1969, p 244.
10. **Ohishi, S.**, *Development of Tea Manufacture in Japan (in Japanese)*, Nousangyoson Bunka Kyokai, Tokyo, 1983.
11. **Tsushida, T.**, Clarification of amino acids metabolism in tea leaves and development of new type tea (Gabaron-tea), *Tea Res. J.*, **72**, 43, 1990.
12. **Matsuura, T., Kakuda, T., Kinoshita, T., Takeuchi, N., and Sasaki, K.**, Theanine formation by tea suspension cells, *Biosci. Biotech. Biochem.*, **56**, 1519, 1994.
13. **Takihara, T., Matsuura, T., Sakane, I., Kakuda, T., Kinoshita, T., and Takeuchi, N.**, Effects of plant growth regulators and carbon sources on theanine formation in callus culture of tea (*Camellia sinensis*), *Biosci. Biotech. Biochem.*, **58**, 1519, 1994.

14. **Kawagishi, H. and Sugiyama, K,** Facile and large-scale synthesis of L-theanine, *Biosci. Biotech. Biochem.*, **56**, 687, 1992.
15. **Yamada, T., Shiode, J.-I., and Tachiki, T.,** Glutaminase of *Pseudomonas nitroreducens*: properties and utilization in synthesis of gamma-glutamyl derivatives, *Annual Reports of IC Biotech.*, **13**, 351, 1990.
16. **Abelian, V. A., Okubo, T., Shamtsian, M. M., Mutoh, K., Chu, D.-C., Kim, M., and Yamamoto, T.,** A novel method of production of theanine by immobilized *Pseudomonas nitroreducens* cells, *Biosci. Biotech. Biochem.*, **57**, 481, 1993.
17. **Tachiki, T., Suzuki, H., Wakisaka, S., Yano, T., and Tochikura, T.,** Production of γ-glutamylmethylamide and glutamylethylamide by coupling of baker's yeast preparations and bacterial glutamine synthetase, *J. Gen. Appl. Microbiol.*, **32**, 545, 1986.
18. **Kimura, R. and Murata, T.,** Effect of theanine on norepinephrine and serotonin levels in rat brain, *Chem. Pharm. Bull.*, **34**, 3053, 1986.
19. **Yokogoshi, H., Kato, Y., Sagesaka, Y. M., Takihara-Matsuura, T., Kakuda, T., and Takeuchi, N.,** Reduction effect of theanine on blood pressure and brain 5-hydroxyindoles in spontaneously hypertensive rats, *Biosci. Biotech. Biochem.*, **59**, 615, 1995.
20. **Kimura, R. and Murata, T.,** Influence of alkylamides of glutamic acid and related compounds on the central nervous system. I. Central depressant effect of theanine, *Chem. Pharm. Bull.*, **19**, 1257, 1971.
21. **Furukawa, S., Kamo, I., Furukawa, Y., Akazawa, S., Satoyoshi, E., Itoh, K., and Hayashi, K.,** A highly sensitive enzyme immunoassay for mouse β-nerve growth factor, *J. Neurochem.*, **40**, 734, 1983.
22. **Matsui, K., Furukawa, S., Shibasaki, H., and Kikuchi, T.,** Reduction of nerve growth factor level in the brain of genetically ataxic mice (weaver, reeler), *FEBS Lett.*, **276**, 78, 1990.

Chapter 13

GREEN TEA EXTRACT AS A REMEDY FOR DIARRHEA IN FARM-RAISED CALVES

N. Ishihara and S. Akachi

TABLE OF CONTENTS

I. Introduction
II. Effects of Administration of Green Tea Extract on Milk-Suckling Calves
    A. Method of Examination
    B. Analysis on Intestinal Microflora
    C. Results Obtained and Their Implication
        1. Convalesce from Diarrhea
        2. Changes in Intestinal Microflora
References

I. INTRODUCTION

Our research group has reported that green tea extract selectively regulates the growth of clostridial bacteria among various intestinal microorganisms [1, 2]. It was also found that green tea extract was effective establishing and maintaining human intestinal microflora in an ideal balanced state [3].

For the calves at rearing farms, diarrhea and pneumonia are the most prevalent diseases and the protection from these diseases is one of the most important tasks in managing the rearing of calves for milking cows. The diseases prevalent in calves during the period of one week to one month after being transferred to a rearing farm are not only the malignant infectious microorganisms but are also caused by the stress from the change in their environment.

We surveyed 75 calves suffering from diarrhea at a rearing farm and investigated the cause. The diarrhea observed for 6 calves was caused by bacterial infection, 10, due to viruses; 9, due to parasites infection; while the other 50, by reasons besides infectious microorganisms.

We examined the effect of green tea extract on calves suffering from diarrhea of non-infectious type and demonstrated that green tea extract exhibits a distinct effect in curing or suppressing diarrhea [4].

II. EFFECTS OF ADMINISTRATION OF GREEN TEA EXTRACT ON MILK-SUCKLING CALVES

A. METHOD OF EXAMINATION

Dried green tea leaves were soaked into 10 weights of boiling water and stirred for 5 min. The mixture was subjected to a filterpress, and the filtrate was spray-dried (Table 1 and Figure 1, a commercial preparation "TEAPECUS^{R}B", Taiyo Kagaku Co., Ltd.) was prepared. A pulverized preparation of the tea extract was mixed with starter and given to calves.

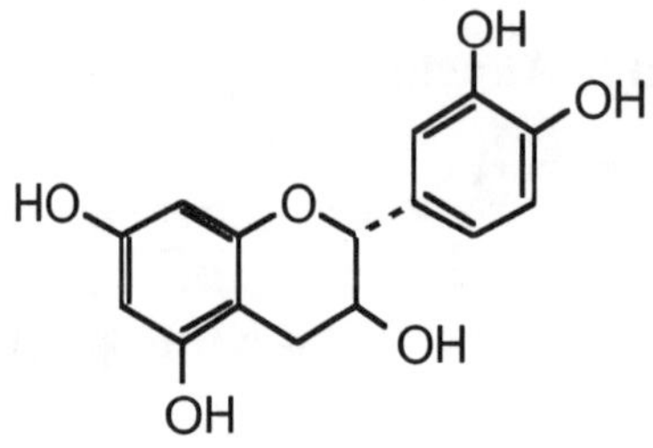

(+)-Catechin

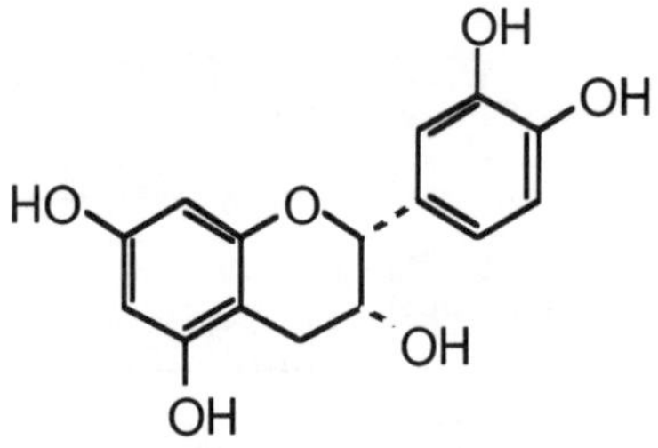

(-)-Epicatechin

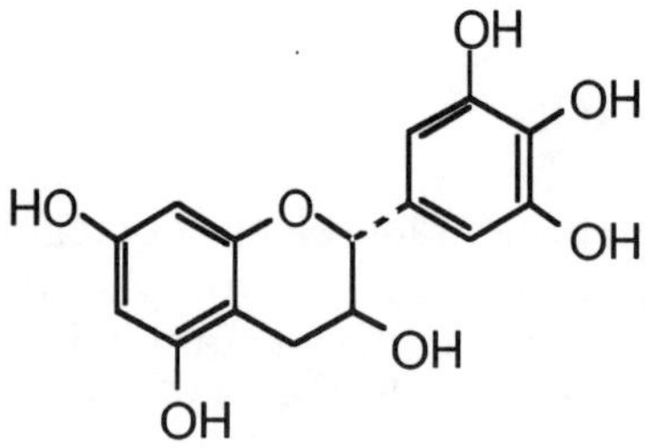

(+)-Gallocatechin

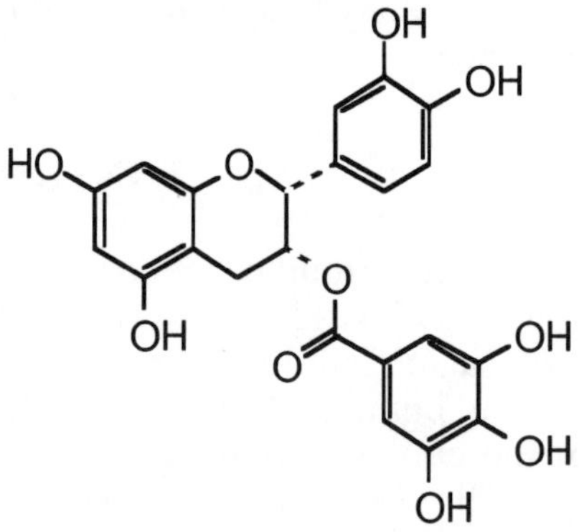

(-)-Epicatechin gallate

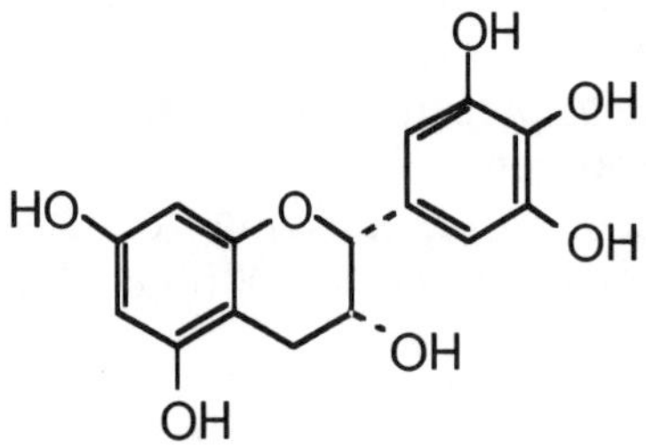

(-)-Epigallocatechin

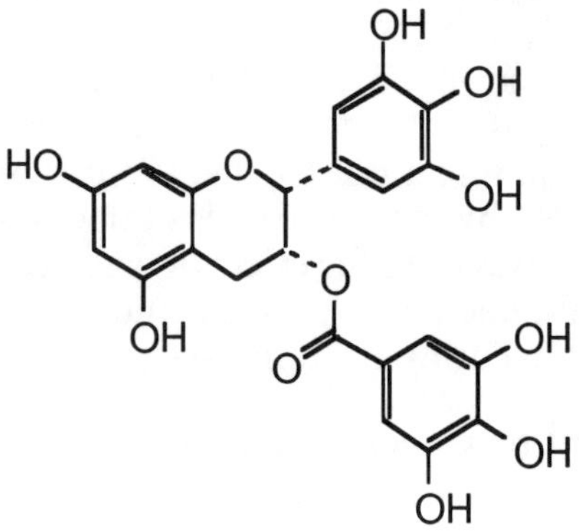

(-)-Epigallocatechin gallate

Figure 1. Main polyphenolic compounds in TEAPECUS [R] B.

Table 1
Characteristics of TEAPECUS^R B

Parameter	Value
Appearance	Brownish yellow powder
Moisture	<6%
Ash	<16%
Polyphenols*	>20%
Reducing sugar as glucose	13.0-14.0%
Total sugar content	30.0-31.0%
Amino groups as glutamic acid	2.0-3.0%

*(-)-gallocatechin > (-)-epigallocatechin > (-)-epigallocatechin gallate > (+)-catechin > (-)-epicatechin > (-)-epicatechingallate

Twenty calves of 10 to 30 days old suffering from diarrhea of non-infectious type, were divided into two groups: 10 calves as the test group and the other 10, as the control group. Calves in the test group were given 1.5 g of the green tea extract (TEAPECUS^{R}B) by mixing with starter, once a day for four weeks. The feces from each calf were inspected every day for scoring the degree of diarrhea according to the following criteria: normal feces, 0; soft, 1; muddy, 2; and watery, 3. The scores were treated by equations shown below, and the incidence of diarrhea or the degree were calculated:

$$\text{Average score of feces} = \frac{\text{Total scores of feces}}{\text{Total days inspected}} \times 100 \quad (1)$$

$$\text{Incidence of diarrhea} = \frac{\text{Total days sufferred from diarrhea}}{\text{Total days inspected}} \times 100 \quad (2)$$

$$\text{Rate of diarrhea suppressed} = \frac{(a) - \text{Total scores of test group}}{\text{Total scores of control group}} \times 100 \quad (3)$$

(a) = Total scores of control group

B. ANALYSIS OF INTESTINAL MICROFLORA

The feces obtained from each calf by mechanical stimulation of the anus before and after administration of the tea extract at 1, 2, 3, and 4 weeks was analyzed by the method of Mitsuoka et al. for microflora using the culture media shown in Table 2 [5, 6].

Table 2
Culture Media and Analytical Method for Intestinal Bacteria

Medium	Main microorganisms enumerated	Degree of dilution for plating[1]	Incubation time (days)
Aerobic culture			
TS blood agar	Predominant aerobes	$10^{-4,-5,-6}$	2
DHL agar	Enterobacteriaceae	$10^{-1,-3,-5,-6}$	2
TATAC agar	*Streptococcus* spp.	$10^{-1,-3,-5,-6}$	2
PEES agar	*Straphylococcus* spp.	$10^{-1,-3,-5,-6}$	2
Anaerobic culture[2]			
EG agar	Predominant anaerobes	$10^{-4,-5,-6}$	3
BL agar	Predominant anaerobes	$10^{-1,-3,-5,-6}$	3
NBGT agar	Bacteroidaceae	$10^{-1,-3,-5,-6}$	3
BS agar	*Bifidobacterium* spp.	$10^{-1,-3,-5,-6}$	3
ES agar	*Eubacterium* spp.	$10^{-1,-3,-5,-6}$	3
VS agar	*Veillonella* spp.	$10^{-1,-3,-5,-6}$	3
LBS agar	*Lactobacillus* spp.	$10^{-1,-3,-5,-6}$	3
CW agar	*Clostridium perfrigens* *Clostridium* spp.	$10^{-1,-3,-5,-6}$	3

[1] 0.5 ml of sample after diluting as indicated was plated on each medium.
[2] Each medium was in a steel wool jar filled with 100% CO_2. TS = trypticase soy (BBL); DHL = deoxycholate hydrogen sulfide-lactose; TATAC = triphenylaterazoliumazide-thallous sulfate-acridine orange crystal violet; PEES = phenylethyl alcohol-egg yolk- *Staphylococcus* no. 110 (EIKEN); EG = Eggerth Gagnon; BL = glucose-blood-liver; NBGT = neomycin-brilliantgreen-taurocholate-bold; BS = *Bifidobacterium* selective; ES = *Eubacterium* Selective; VS = *Veillonella* selective; LBS = *Lactobacillus* selective (BBL); CW = *Clostridium perfrigens* selective-egg yolk (Nissui)

A serial dilution (10^{-1} to 10^{-6}) of the fecal specimens was made using anaerobic diluent, mixing thoroughly. Aliquots of the diluted samples were taken and spread onto an agar plate of the medium mentioned above and incubated at 37°C for 3 days under CO_2 atmosphere. Bacterial colonies on the respective medium were counted and identified according to their colonial and cellular morphologies (for Gram staining, spore formation, and aerobic growth). The bacterial cell counts per gram of wet feces were expressed as a logarithm value. The analytical data obtained were criticized by applying the Student's t-test for significance.

C. RESULTS OBTAINED AND THEIR IMPLICATION

1. Convalesce from diarrhea

As shown in Table 3, the incidence of diarrhea observed in the test group was 11.6%, while that of the control group was 49.7% with a significance level of 1.0%. A similar result was obtained from the fecal score showing that the control group was 35.5, while that of the test group was 12.5 with a significance level of 1.0%. These results clearly indicate that administration of the tea extract is effective to cure or suppress the degree of diarrhea which occurrs non-infectiously in calves.

Table 3

Effect of Oral Admistration
of TEAPECUS^R B on Diarrhea in Nursing Calves

	Test Group	Control Group
Incidence of diarrhea (%)	11.6	49.7
Fecal score (point)	12.5	39.5

2. Changes in intestinal microflora

Figure 2 (a) and (b) shows the changes in cellular counts of several intestinal bacteria.

As can be seen from Figure 2 (a) and (b), the total bacterial cell counts decreased with an increase in the feeding period of calves in both groups. However, a significant difference in the rate of the decrease was observed between the two groups. The rate of decrease of *Bifidobacterium* and *Lactobacillus* was much slower in the test group than the control group. On the other hand, the decreasing rate of *Clostridium perfringens* was faster in the test group than in the control group.

The cell counts of *Staphylococcus, Streptococcus, Eubacterium,* and Bacteroidaceae also decreased, but no significant difference in the decreasing rates was observed between the two groups.

The results above indicate that the green tea polyphenols were stimulative for the growth of *Bifidobacterium* and *Lactobacillus* which are useful intestinal bacteria. On the other hand, the polyphenols suppressed the growth of

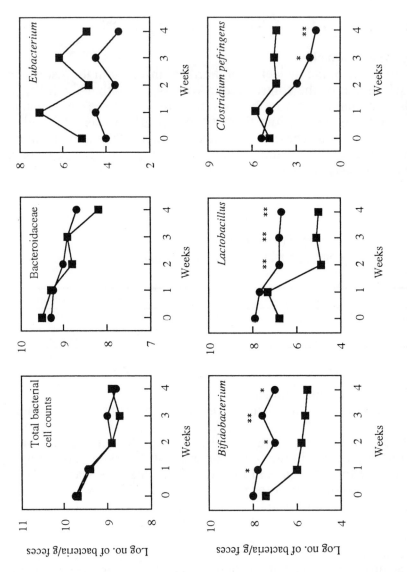

Figure 2 (a). Effects of oral administration of TEAPECUS^R B on intestinal bacteria in nursing calves. Significance for; *, p<0.05; **, p<0.01 ■——, Control group; ●——, test group.

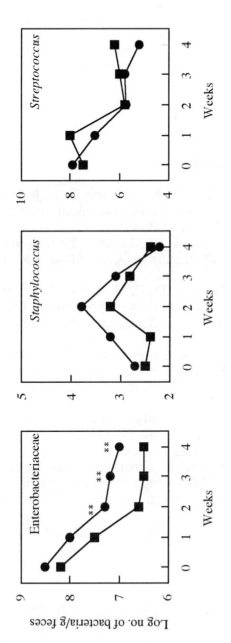

Figure 2 (b). Effects of oral administration of TEAPECUS^R B on intestinal bacteria in nursing calves. Significance for; *, p<0.05; **, p<0.01
■——■, Control group; ●——●, test group.

Clostridium perfringens which is considered to be harmful. It has been reported that the occurrence of imbalance in the intestinal microflora causes a reduction of immunity and feed efficiency, leading the host animal to be sensitive to pathogenic microorganisms or non-pathogenic diarrhea [7].

The calves used in the test above were those brought from various places to the collective rearing farms. Due to change of environment, they were liable to suffer from diarrhea due to stress and nervousness.

The application of green tea extracts by the method described above is now gradually spreading in Japan not only for calves, but also for milking cows. We emphasize here that the leftover fraction remaining after removal of polyphenols from TEAPECUS^{R}B did not show any effect for suppressing the diarrhea on calves.

REFERENCES

1. **Ahn, Y.-J., Sakanaka, S., Kim, M., Kawamura, T., Fujisawa, M., and Mitsuoka, T.,** Effect of green tea extract on growth of intestinal bacteria, *Microb. Ecol. in Health and Disease*, **3**, 335, 1990.
2. **Ahn, Y.-J., Kawamura, T., Kim, M., and Yamamoto, T.,** Tea polyphenols: Selective growth inhibitors of *Clostridium spp.*, *Agric. Biol. Chem.*, **55**, 1425, 1991.
3. **Okubo, T., Ishihara, N., Oura, A., Serit, M., Kim, M., Yamamoto, T., and Mitsuoka, T.,** *In Vivo* effects of tea polyphenol intake on human intestinal microflora and metabolism, *Biosci. Biotech. Biochem.*, **56**, 588, 1992.
4. **Ishihara, N., Mamiya, S., Aoi, N., Yamade, T., Nakanishi, K., Akachi, S., Fujiki, M., and Kim, M.,** The effect of green tea extracts for calves suffering from diarrhea of non-infectious type, *Anim. Husbundry (in Japanese)*, **50**, 275, 1996.
5. **Mitsuoka, T., Sega, S., and Yamamoto, S.,** Eine verbesserte methodik der qualitativen und quantitativen analyse der darm flora von menschen und tieren, *Hyg. I Abt. Org.*, **A195**, 455, 1965.
6. **Mitsuoka, T., Ohno, K., Benno, Y., Suzuki, K., and Namba, K.,** Die faekalflora bei menschen. IV. Mitteilung: Vergleich des neu entwickelten verfahrens mit dem bisherigen ublichen verfahren zur darmflora analyse, *Hyg. I Abt. Org.*, **A234**, 219, 1976.
7. **Mitsuoka, T.,** Recent trends in research on intestinal flora, *Bifidobacteria Microflora*, **1**, 3, 1982.

TABLES OF DATA ON THE ANTIMICROBIAL ACTIVITIES OF GREEN TEA EXTRACTS

S. Sakanaka, T. Okubo, S. Akachi, K. Mabe, and M. Matsumoto

Table 1
Antimicrobial Activity of Green Tea Extracts[1]

Microorganisms examined	Minimum inhibitory concentration (µg/ml) [2]
Bacteria	
Escherichia coli IFO 3545	2,000
Escherichia coli IFO 3301	1,800
Escherichia coli O-157: H7 Sakai[3]	250
Escherichia coli O-157: H7 ATCC 43895	250
Proteus vulgaris IFO 3581	300
Pseudomonas aeruginosa IFO 3080	4,000
Pseudomonas fluorescens IFO 13922	2,000
Serratia marcescens IFO 3046	600
Bacillus subtilis IFO 3007	700
Bacillus cereus ATCC 14579	600
Bacillus brevis IFO 3331	800
Bacillus circulans IFO 13626	900
Bacillus macerans JCM 2500	500
Bacillus polymyxa JCM 2507	1,000
Staphylococcus aureus IFO 12732	2,000
Lactobacillus acidophilis IAM 1043	1,000
Streptococcus lactis IFO 12546	500
Streptococcus mutans IFO 13955	1,000
Streptococcus mutans MT 8148	500
Streptococcus mutans 6715 DP	500
Helicobacter pylori ATCC 43504	600
Propionibacterium acnes ATCC 6919	500
Propionibacterium acnes ATCC 11828	500
Prophyromonas gingvalis ATCC 33277	500

Fungi / Yeast
The growth of the fungi and yeasts given with the following were not affected even at the concentration of 4,000 µg of green tea extract per ml media: *Saccharomyces cerevisiae* IFO 0203, *Candida albicans* IFO 1061, *Rhodotorula rubra* IFO 0001, *Hansenula anomala* IFO 0136, *Kluyveromyces fragilis* IFO 1963, *Kluyveromyces lactis* IFO1090, *Metschnikowia pulcherrima* IFO 1678, *Aspergillus niger* ATCC 3275, *Mucor mucedo* IFO 7684, *Rhizopus chinensis* IFO 4745, *Penicillium chrysogenum* IFO 5809, *Penicillium citrinum* IFO 7784, *Trycophyton rubrum* IFO 5807, *Trycophyton mentagrophytes* IFO 5466, *Trycophyton mentagrophytes* IFO 5809, and *Trycophyton tonsurans* IFO 5946.

[1] As the green tea extract, "Sunphenon^R" (Taiyo Kagaku Co., Ltd.) was used which was prepared by the method described in Chapter 3.

[2] For measurement of the minimum inhibitory concentration (MIC), 0.1 ml of the green tea extracts of which concentrations were varied by serial dilution was added to 9.9 ml of medium containing 1.5% agar at about 60°C in a petri dish. The mixture was agitated thoroughly and solidified at 37°C. One platinum loop of the microorganism suspension obtained by preculture was inoculated on the agar medium and incubated at 37°C for 48 hr for bacteria or at 25°C for 96 hr for fungi and yeasts.
Growth medium: brain heart infusion (BHI, DIFCO Laboratories) for bacteria and malt extract broth (BBL Microbiology Systems) for fungi and yeasts.

[3] The secretion of verotoxin by the bacterium has been reported to be inhibited by 50 µg green tea extract per ml (Konishi et al., Ann. Meeting of Jap. Soc. for Biosci. Biotech. Biochem. (in Japanese), p 52, 1997, Tokyo).

Table 2

Growth Inhibition Thermophilic Spore-Forming Bacteria by Green Tea Extracts

Bacteria examined	Minimum inhibitory concentration (μg/ml)
Bacillus stearothermophilus IAM 1035	100
Bacillus stearothermophilus IFO 12550	150
Bacillus stearothermophilus ATCC 12980	150
Bacillus coagulans JCM2257	200
Clostridium thermoaceticum No 5801	400
Clostridium thermoaceticum No 5802	400
Clostridium thermoaceticum No 5809	400
Clostridium thermosaccharolyticum No 5604	100

Growth medium: brain heart infusion (BHI, DIFCO Laboratories) and the modified thioglycollate medium (1.7% trypticase, 0.3% phytone, 0.6% glucose, 0.25% NaCl, 0.05% Na-thioglycollate, 0.025% L-cystine, and 0.01% Na_2SO_3); culture condition, aerobically for Bacillus stearothermophilus (50°C, 48 hr), Bacillus coagulans (37°C, 48 hr), and anaerobically for Clostridium bacteria (55°C, 3 days).

Table 3

Effect of Green Tea Extracts on the D-Value of Bacillus stearothermophilus

	D-value (min)*		
	115°C	120°C	125°C
Control	18.3	4.0	2.0
Green tea extracts (500 ppm)	10.0	2.2	0.5

The spores of Bacillus stearothermophilus IFO 12550 were obtained by culturing in the spore forming medium (0.5% polypeptone, 0.1% glucose, 0.3% yeast extract, 0.2% NaCl, 0.05% $MnSO_4$, and 2.0% agar, pH 7.2) at 55.5°C for 3 days. The spore suspension prepared by centrifuging the culture, washing with M/15 phosphate pH 7.0, and adjusting the spore concentration at 1.1×10^6 CFU/ml was heated in a glass tube (7 × 100 mm) at the temperatures indicated.

*D value: the heating time (min) required for 10% decrease of CFU of spores.

Table 4

Growth Inhibition of Various Fish Pathogens by Green Tea Extract

Host fish and microorganisms	Minimum inhibitory concentration (µg/ml)[1]
Ayu	
Vibrio anguillarum IFO13266	200
Vibrio anguillarum UP-1	200
Vibrio anguillarum PT-213	150
Vibrio anguillarum PT-493	150
Vibrio spp.	200
Vibrio spp.	200
Crawfish	
Vibrio sp. PJ	50
Vibrio alguillarum	400
Vibrio fluvialis	200
Vibrio damsela ATCC 33539	200
Yellowtail	
Streptococcus spp.	1,000
Streptococcus spp.	800
Streptococcus KS-8903	700
Streptococcus KS-8930	800
Streptococcus KS-8982	900
Streptococcus β-hemlosys	900
Pasteurella piscicida spp.	100
Pasteurella piscicida OT-8447	200
Pasteurella piscicida 5866	150
Eel	
Edwardsiella tarda SH-89133	400
Edwardsiella tarda E-2812	300
Edwardsiella tarda SY-84006	400
Vibrio vulnificus ATCC 33147	200
Vibrio parahaemolyticus ATCC 17802	200
Salmon	
Vibrio vulnificus	200
Vibrio spp.	100
Vibrio spp.	150
Other fish	
Aeromonas salmonisida	800
Aeromonas hydrophila	200
Vibrio alguillarum ATCC 19264	400
Vibrio harveyi	100

[1]The examination method was the same as those applied in Table 1. Growth medium of bacteria was brain heart infusion (BHI, DIFCO Laboratories) containing 1.5% NaCl.

Table 5

Growth Inhibition of Various Animal Pathogens by Green Tea Extract

Host aminal and microorganisms	Minimum inhibitory concentration (μg/ml)[1]
Cattle	
Salmonella dublin L-729	4,000
Pseudomonas aeruginosa KK-1001	500
Staphylococcus aureus KK103	500
Staphylococcus aureus spp.	1,000
Staphylococcus aureus KK101	1,000
Staphylococcus aureus ATCC 25923[2]	100
Staphylococcus epidermidis KK108	500
Staphylococcus epidermidis spp.	500
Escherichia coli K99	>4,000
Pig	
Salmonella enteritidis ZK2a	4,000
Escherichia coli K88 (Abbotstown)	4,000
Escherichia coli K88 (G1253)	4,000
Escherichia coli K88 (MN-1)	4,000
Chicken	
Salmonella enteritidis L-58	4,000
Salmonella typhimurium L-413	4,000
Salmonella infantis L-164	4,000
Salmonella thompson L-131	4,000
Salmonella sofia L-59	2,000
Salmonella mbandaka L-743	4,000
Salmonella mbandaka spp.	4,000
Salmonella huderberg spp.	4,000

[1] The examination method was the same as those mentioned in Table 1.
[2] Methicillin resistant *Staphylococcus aureus* (MRSA) strain.

INDEX

A

Absolute configuration	25, 30
Absorption of polyphenols	53
Acetic acid	25, 115, 116
Acetonitrile	24, 25
Acid forming bacteria	109, 115
Actinomyces viscosus	103
Active oxygen species	75
Adduct	
polyphenol-carcinogen	69
Adenine	
diet	76, 80, 81
induced chronic renal failure	76
Adenovirus	118
Adherence	
buccal epithelial cells	104
glass surface	91
tooth surface	88, 91, 94
Administration	51-53, 56
Adrenal glands	53
Aeromonas hydrophila	148
Aeromonas salmonisida	148
Aging	109
Amino acid	23
cysteine	37
theanine	23
glutamic acid	18
γ-Aminobutyric acid	18, 19
Ammonia	116, 117, 125
Amylase	53
Animal pathogens	149
Antagonist	134
Antibacterial activities	
of green tea extracts	110, 146-149
Antibiotics	56
Anticaries effect	37
Antidecoloring effect	39-41
Antimutagenicity	110
Antioxidant	
chain-breaking	76
Antioxidative activity	37, 110
Antitumor	110
Antiviral	118
Araliaceae	109
Arenavirus	118
Arylhydrocarbonhydroxylase	70
L-Ascorbate	40
Aspergillus niger	146
Asymmetric carbon atoms	23
Average score of feces	139
Ayu	148
2,2'-Azobis (2-aminopropane) hydrochloride (AAAPH)	44
2,2'-Azobis [2-methylpropanenitrile]	42
Azoxymethane	53

B

Bacillus	
brevis	146
cereus	146
circulans	146
coagulans	147
macerans	146
polymyxa	146
spp.	113
stearothermophilus	147
subtilis	146
Bacteria	
Clostridium genera	70
Bacteroidaceae	113, 114, 140-142
Bacteroides	
distasonis	111
fragilis	110, 111
thetaiotaomicron	111
vulgatus	111
Benzo(*a*)pyrene (BP)	64

Benzopyrenediolepoxide		bladder	63
(BPDE)	65	breast	63
Beverage	40	colon	63-69
Bifidobacterium		chemoprevention	61-73
adolescentis	110, 111	duodenum	64
bifidum	111	esophagus	63, 64
breve	110, 111	forestomach	64
infantis	110, 111	glandular stomach	64
longum	110, 111	kidney	63
spp.	113-115, 140,	large intestine	66
selective medium	140	liver	63, 65
Bile	56	lung	63, 65
Biliary excretion	54	mammary gland	65
Bilirubin	76	nasopharynx	63
Biosynthetic pathway		pancreas	63, 65
of catechin	16	rectum	63
BL agar	140	risk	62
Black tea	42, 46, 87	skin	65
Blood pressure	51, 52, 133	small intestine	64
Bone marrow	53	stomach	63
Brain	53	urinary tract	63
brain heart infusion (BHI)	146-148	uterus	63
brain wave	133	Cancer prevention	51
Brucella agar	111	*Candida albicans*	146
BS agar	140	Canola oil	42
Bunyavirus	118	Caproic acid	116
Butylated hydroxytoluene		Carbohydrate	20
(BHT)	42, 46	Carcinogenesis	46, 61, 65
Butyric acid	116	Cardiovascular disease	52
		Caries score	95, 98
		Cariogenesis	61, 65
C		Cariogenic bacteria	
		minimum inhibitory	
		concentrations (MIC)	89
Caffeine	1, 2, 15, 17, 23, 24, 33, 42, 110	Cariogenicity	
		effects of tea	
		polyphenols	89
Calicivirus	118		
Calves		Carotenoids	
rearing farms of	137	β-carotene	39-41, 76
milk sucking	137	Catalase	76
Camellia		Catechin	37, 42, 46
C. grocilipes	2	(+)-catechin (C)	23, 25-27, 29, 30, 33, 34, 42-45, 53-57, 78, 110, 112
C. irrawadiensis	2		
C. pubicosta	2		
C. sinensis			
((L) O. Kuntze)	1, 2		
C. taliensis	2	(-)-epicatechin (EC)	42, 43, 45, 54, 55, 110, 112
Cancer			

(-)-epigallocatechin (EGC)	42, 45, 55, 110, 112	*paraputrificum*	111
		perfringens	109-114, 140-142, 144
(-)-epicatechin-3-gallate (ECg)	42, 43, 45, 110, 112	*perfringens* selective-egg yolk	140
(+)-gallocatechin (GC)	45, 110, 112	*ramosum*	110, 111, 113-115, 140, 142
(-)-epigallocatechin-3-gallate (EGCg)	42, 44, 45, 112	spp.	
[U-^{14}C]catechin	53, 54, 56	*thermoaceticum*	147
Cattle	149	*thermosaccharolyticum*	147
Ceruloplasmin	76	Cold tolerance of tea plant	4
Chemical carcinogen		Colon cancer	53
azoxymethane (AOM)	65-68	Coronavirus	118
7,12-dimethylbenzanthracene (DMBA)	65	*Corynebacterium*	113
		Coxsackie virus B6	118
		Crawfish	148
N-methyl-N'-nitro-N-nitrosoguanidine (MNNG)	64	Creatinine	78
		Creatol	78
		Cresol	116
4-methylnitrosoamino-3-pyridyl-butanone (NNK)	65	Cultivation	1, 2, 6
		Curved rods	113, 114
		CW agar	140
4-nitroquinoline-1-oxide	65	Cyclodextrins	24, 34
N-nitroso-bis(2-oxopropyl)amine (BOP)	65	β-cyclodextrin (β-CDx)	34
		β-CD polymer	17
N-nitrosodiethylamine (NDEA)	64, 65	Cysteine	33, 34
		Cytochrome P-450	70
N-nitrosomethylbenzylamine (NMBzA)	64		
phorbol ester	70	**D**	
12-O-tetradecanoylphorbol-1,3-acetate (TPA)	65	*ddy* mice	57
Chemical components of tea	2, 9	Decaffeination	17
Chemical shift	29, 30, 34	Dental caries	52
Chicken	53, 149	epidemiological study	97
Cholecystokinin	53, 54	in rats	94
Cholesterol	46, 117	Deodorant	126
Circular dichroism	34	Deodorizing effect	123
Citric acid	42	Deoxycholate hydrogen sulfide-lactose	140
Clostridia	109, 110, 112, 114	DHL agar	140
Clostridium	106	Diaion HP-20	24
bifermentans	111	Diarrhea	
butyricum	110, 111	convalesce from	141
coccoides	110, 111	degree of	141
difficile	109, 111, 112	incidence of	141
		in nursing calves	141
innocuum	111	non-pathogenic	144

observations	137	(-)-Epigallocatechin, (-)-EGC	23, 25-27, 29-31, 78, 89, 106
Diarylpropan-2-ol metabolites	57		
Digestibility	53		
Digestive tracts	51, 53, 118	(-)-Epigallocatechin-3-(3"-O-methylgalate)	26, 33
2,8-Dihydroxyadenine	76		
Dimeric flavan-3-ol gallates	25	(-)-Epigallocatechin-p-coumaroate	25
Dimeric proanthocyanin gallates	25	(-)-Epigallocatechin digallate	25
1,2-Dimethylhydrazine	47	(-)-Epigallocatechin gallate, (-)-EGCg	23, 24, 25-27, 29-31, 33-35, 78, 89, 92, 93, 106, 119
Dimethyl sulfide	124		
1,1-Diphenyl-2-picrylhydrazyl (DPPH)	42		
Distribution of administrated polyphenols	51, 53		
DNA	43, 46, 47		
polymerase	118	adherence inhibition	106
DNA virus	118	urinary methylguanidine	80, 81
Dose	51-53, 54	Epimerization	34
Dough noodle	39	Epinephrine	133
D-value	147	Epithelial cells	106, 107
		ES agar	140
		Escherichia coli	110, 111, 146, 152
E			
		K99	149
Edwardsiella tarda	148	K88	149
Eel	148	O-157: H Sakai	146
EG agar	140	O-157: H ATCC43895	146
Eggerth Gagnon	140	Ester ratio	117
Electrophilic specimens	23	7-Ethoxycoumari-*N-O*-deethylase	70
Enzymation	1, 2		
Enterovirus	118	Ethylacetate	23-25, 89
Enterobacteria	114	Ethylamine	133, 134
Enterobacteriaceae	113, 140, 143	4-Ethylphenol	116
		Eubacterium	
Enzyme		*aerofaciens*	111
activities of feces	117	*lentum*	110, 111
(-)-Epicatechin, (-)-EC	23, 29, 30, 31, 33, 34, 78, 89, 105	*imosum*	111
		spp.	113, 114, 140-142
(-)-Epicatechin-3-(3"-O-methylgallate)	26, 33	selective medium	140
		Excretion	
(-)-Epicatechin gallate, (-)-ECg	23, 25-27, 29-31, 33, 78, 89, 92, 93, 106, 119	biliary excretion	54
		F	
effect on serum constituents	82	Fecal pH	115
		Fecal score	141
Epidemiological study	62-64	Feces	51, 56

enzyme activities of	115, 117	Green tea	42, 46
pH value of	115	Green tea infusion	23, 51
$FeCl_3$	31	Green tea polyphenols (GTP)	23-25, 29-31, 51, 52, 53, 56
Fermentability	4		
Fermentation	1, 6		
Ferric ion	69	growth inhibition of *Porphyromonas gingivalis*	104
Ferritin	76		
Fish disease bacteria	148		
Fissure caries lesions	94	prevention of dental caries	87-89, 97
Flavi virus	118	Growth factor	133
Fluoride	19, 20, 87, 97	Guanidinosuccinic acid	76
		Guinea pig	54
Formation constant	34	Gut tube	56
Free cholesterol	117	Gyokuro	110
Free radicals	75	Gyorgy	
Fried noodle	39	broth	110
		medium	111

G

H

Gallic acid	23, 31, 119		
ester	23, 33	Haemagglutination activity	118
(+)-Gallocatechin, (+)-GC	23, 25-27, 29, 30, 33, 78, 106	Halitosis	124, 126
		Hansenula anomala	146
		HDL-cholesterol	51, 117
(-)-Gallocatechin gallate, (-)-GCg	23, 25-27, 29, 30, 78, 106	Heart	53
		Helicobacter pylori	146
		Hemodialysis patients	82
		Hepadna virus	118
Gel filtration	34	Hepatocarcinogen	47
Gelatin	31	Hepatoma	65
Ginseng extract	109	Herpes simplex virus	118
Glucan		Herpes virus	118
water-insoluble	88	Heteropolysaccharides	109
Glucose	53	Hetrocyclic amine (HCA)	70
Glucose-blood-liver	140	Hexahydroxydiphenic acid	23
β-Glucosidase	117	High performance liquid chromatography (HPLC)	24-26
Glucosyltransferase			
inhibitory effects of tea polyphenols	91	High porosity polystyrene gel	24, 25
		HIV-reverse transcriptase	37, 119
β-Glucuronidase	117	Human immunodeficiency virus (HIV)	118
Glucuronide	55, 57		
L-glutamate ethylamine ligase	134	Hybrid	4
		Hydrogen	34
Glutamic oxaloacetic transaminase (GOT)	46	bonding	33
		peroxide	43
Glutamic pyruvic transaminase (GPT)	46	sulfide	124
		Hydrophobic effects	33
Glutathione peroxidase	43, 76	Hydrophobic interaction	33

Hydroxy radicals	43, 75	**L**	
8-Hydroxydeoxyguanosine (8-OHdG)	46, 47	*Lactobacillus*	
Hydroxylation pattern	25, 30	acidophilus	111, 146
Hyperlipemia	46	casei	110, 111
Hyperlipidemia	51, 52	salivarius	110, 111
Hypertension	51	selective medium	140
Hypocholesterolemia	51	spp.	113, 114, 140, 142
Hypolipemic	110	Lactoferrin	76
		Lard oil	37-39
I		Large intestine	56
		LBS agar	140
Immobilized cell	135, 136	Lethal dose	56
Incidence of diarrhea	139	Lipid	20
Indole	116	peroxide	43, 46
Influenza		β-Lipoprotein	117
virus A	118	Lipoprotein	46
virus B	118	Liposome	43
Infusion	13, 14	Liver	53
Initiation	61	Low density lipoprotein (LDL)	46
Intestinal bacteria		Lung	53
analysis of	137		
culture media and method	140		
Intestinal microflora		**M**	
analysis of	137		
changes in	137, 141	Madin-Darby canine kidney (MDCK) cells	118
ecology of	110	Malic acid	42
Intestinal microoranism	56	Malignant neoplasm	61
growth inhibition of	110	Malt extract broth	146
growth response of	110	Margarine	40
Intestine	51, 53, 56	Mass spectrometry (MS)	24
intestinal wall	56	Matcha	7, 9
small intestine	53	Maximum absorption wave-length	29
Iron	53	*Megasphaera*	113, 114
Isosbestic point	34	*Melaphis chinensis*	98
Isotope	51	Melting point	29
		Metabolic fate	51
K		Metabolic pathway	51, 56, 57
		Metabolism	51, 54
Kidney	53, 75	Metabolites	51, 54, 56
Kluyveromyces fragilis	146	Metal chelater	23
Kluyveromyces lactis	146	Metal ion	24
		Methanol	24, 25
		Methanol-d4	29, 30
		δ-(3-methoxy hydroxy phenyl)-γ-valerolactone	57

Methyl mercaptan (CH$_3$SH)	34, 123, 124	**O**	
Methylguanidine	75-85	Oolong tea	42, 46, 87
as uremic toxin	77	Optical rotation	29
formation	78	Organotropism	53
Methylsulfinyl group	34	Origin	1, 4
Metschnikowia pulcherrima	146	Orinithine decarboxylase (ODC)	70
Mice	60		
Micrococcaceae	113	Orthomyxovirus	118
Micrococci	114	Ovary	53
Microflora	56, 57	Oxidation	33, 34
Microorganism	56	Oxidative radical	69
Milk suckling calves	137	Oxidative radicals scavenger	23
Minimum inhibitory concentration (MIC)	146-149	Oxygen	24
		Oxygen radical	69
Molds	113, 114		
Molecular formula	29		
Molecular weight	29, 33	**P**	
Monkey kidney MA 104 cells	118		
Mucor mucedo	146	*Panax ginseng*	109
Muscle	53	Pancreatic enzymes	53
Myricetin	46	Paramyxovirus	118
		Parvovirus	118
		Pasteurella piscicida	148
N		Pathogenic microorganisms	144
NBGT agar	140	non-	144
Neomycin-brilliantgreen-taurocholate-blood	140	viruses	118
		PEES agar	140
Neurotransmitter	137	*Penicillium chrysogenum*	146
2-Nitropropane	47	*Penicillium citrinum*	146
Nitroreductase	117	3,3',4',5,7-Pentahydroxyflavan	23
Nitrosation inhibitor	23	Peptococcaceae	113, 114
N,N-Dimethylformamide	25	Peptone yeast fildes (PYF)	110
Nuclear magnetic resonance (NMR)	24	Periodontal disease	88, 103
		Peroxidase	76
A-ring	29, 32	Peroxide value (PV)	37-39
B-ring	29, 32, 34, 37	Phenol	116
		Phenylethyl alcohol-egg yolk-*Staphylococcus* no. 110	140
^{13}C-NMR	34		
^{13}C-NMR spectra	25, 30	Phloroglucinol reaction	31
C-ring	32	Phosphatidylcholine (PC)	43
3-O-galloyl	29, 32	Photochemical properties	25, 26, 33
^{1}H-NMR	25, 33, 34	Phytone	147
^{1}H-NMR spectra	29	Picorna virus	118
Nucleophilic centers	23	Pig	149
		Plant chemistry	24
		Plaque	88, 89, 96-98, 103, 104

Plasma	53	Radioactivity	53, 54
Poliovirus	118	Rate of diarrhea	139
Polyphenols	1, 2, 4, 13, 15, 23-26, 33, 34, 51-53, 56	Rats	52, 53, 54, 55, 56
		Reaction	
		fenton	69
Polyvinyl alcohol column	89	maillard	70
Polyvinyl pyrrolidone	33	nitrosation	69
Popovavirus	118	Recycling liquid chromatography	24, 25, 27
Porphyromonas gingivalis			
adherence inhibition	104	Relaxation	137
growth inhibition	104	Renal failure	52, 75
minimum inhibitory concentration	104	adenine-induced	76
		Reoviridae	118
Porphyromonas melaninogenicus	104	Reovirus	118
		Respiratory organs	118
Poxvirus	118	Retrovirus	118
Predominant		Reverse transcriptase	118
aerobes	140	Rhabdovirus	118
anaerobes	140	*Rhizopus chinensis*	146
Proanthocyanidins	23	*Rhodotorura rubra*	146
Processing	1, 6, 7	RIKEN culture collection	111
Progression	61	RNA-polymerase	118
Promotion	61	RNA virus	118
Propionibacterium acnes	146		
Propionic acid	115, 116		
Propyl galatte	45		
Prospec dye	96	**S**	
Protein kinase C	70		
Proteus vulgaris	146	*Saccharomyces cerevisiae*	146
Pseudomonas aeruginosa	113, 114, 146, 149	Safranin solution	109
		Salivary gland	53
		Salmon	41, 148
Pseudomonas fluorescens	146	*Salmonella*	
Pseudomonas nitroreducens	135	*dublin*	149
Purification	23-25, 33	*entritidis*	149
Putrefactive products	115, 116	*huderberg*	149
PYF medium	111	*infantis*	149
		mbandaka	149
		sofia	149
Q		*thompson*	149
		typhimurium	149
Quercetin	46	Saponines	110
		SENCAR mice	47
		Sencha	7, 9, 110
R		*Serratia marcescens*	146
		Sesaminol	46
Rabbit blood cell	45	Sexual organ	118
Radical initiator	42, 43	Silica gel column	90
Radical-scavenger	37		

Sister chromatid exchange (SCE)	64	green tea leaves	24, 25, 33
		Tea polyphenol	37, 51-55
Skatole	116	components	89
Skin	53	MIC for cariogenic bacteria	89, 90
Sodium copper chrolophyllin	124-126		
Soybean lipoxygenase	33	prevention of dental caries	87-89, 97
Soybean oil	38, 39		
Spleen	53	suppressive effect of uremic toxin	75-85
Spore forming medium	147		
Staphylococcus	141, 143	scavenging reaction	78
aureus	106, 146	suppression of methyl-guanidine production	83
epidermidis	149		
Streptococcaceae	113	TEAPECUS^{R}B	
Streptococci	114	characteristics of	138
cariogenic	88	oral administration of	142, 143
Streptococcus	106, 140, 141, 143	Testis	53
		12-*O*-Tetradecanoyl-phorbol-13-acetate	47
β-*hemlosys*	148		
lactis	146	Tetramethylsiane	29, 30
mutans	88, 89, 91-93, 95, 146	Thea sinensis L.	110
		Theaceae	1, 5, 10, 110
		Theaflavin	42, 46
piscicida	148	theaflavin digallate	42
salivalius	106	theaflavin monogallate	42
sanguis	106	Theanine	1, 2, 4, 18, 110
sobrinus	89, 91-93		
Structure		γ-amino butyric acid	134
molecular	25-27, 29, 33, 34	biosynthesis	133, 134
		enzymic synthesis	134, 135
Sucrose	88	γ-ethylamino-L-glutamic acid	133
Sulfate	56		
Sulphuric acid	31	metabolism	133, 134
SUNPHENON^R	24, 52, 60	Theasinensin A	25
Superoxide		Theasinensin B	25
dismutase (SOD)	43, 76	Thermophilic spore forming bacteria	147
radical	43		
Synergistic effect	42	Thioglycollate medium modified	147
		Tissue	53
T		Tobacco	125
		Tocopherol	37-39, 42, 45, 46
Tabacco	125		
Tannin	53	Togavirus	118
Tartaric acid	42	Topography	137
TATAC agar	140	Total cholesterol	117
Taxonomy	1-3	Toxicity	51, 56
dualism	4	Transferrin	76
Tea extract	123	Triglyceride	46
Tea leaves	23, 25	Trimethylamine	123, 124

Triphenylaterazoliumazide-thallous sulfate-acridine orange crystal violet	140
Triton X-100	33
Trycophyton mentagrophytes	146
Trycophyton rubrum	146
Trycophyton tonsurans	146
Trypsin	53
Trypticase	147
Trypticase soy	140
TS blood agar	140
Tumor	43, 109
Tumorigenesis	64, 65, 69
Tween	20
Tween 20	33

U

Ubiquinol	76
Ultraviolet ray	65
Uremic toxin formation	75
Uric acid	76
Urine	51, 54, 56
UV spectra	34

V

Vaccination	118
Vaccinia virus	118
Valeric acid	116
Variety of *C. sinensis*	
assamica	2, 5
sinensis	2, 5
Veillonella	
spp.	113, 114, 140
selective medium	140
Vibrio	
anguillarum	148
damsela	148
fluvialis	148
harveyi	148
parahaemolyticus	148
spp.	148
vulnificus	148
Virus infection	118

Vitamin	19, 110
E	43, 76
C	76
Volatile fatty acids	115, 116
VS agar	140

Y

Yeast alcohol dehydrogenase	33
Yeast extract	147
Yeasts	113, 114
Yellow tail	148